Medical Imaging

AN ILLUSTRATED COLOUR TEXT

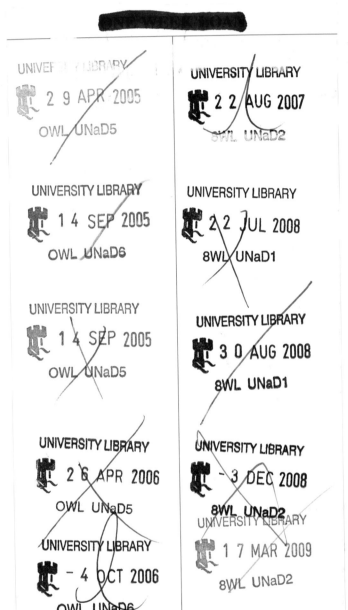

Commissioning Editor: Timothy Horne
Project Development Manager: Siân Jarman
Project Manager: Nancy Arnott
Designer: Erik Bigland
Illustrator: Graeme Chambers

Medical Imaging

AN ILLUSTRATED COLOUR TEXT

Edited by

Peter Renton DMRD FRCR
Consultant Radiologist
Royal National Orthopaedic Hospital,
London, UK

Contributors

Paul Butler
Consultant Neuroradiologist
Royal London Hospital,
London, UK

Steven Halligan
Consultant Radiologist
Northwick Park and St Mark's Hospital
Harrow, Middlesex, UK

Michael Kellett
Formerly Consultant Radiologist
Middlesex Hospital, London, UK

Rakesh Misra
Consultant Radiologist
Wycombe General Hospital
High Wycombe, Buckinghamshire, UK

Michael Rubens
Consultant Radiologist and Consultant
Cardiologist
Royal Brompton and National Heart
Hospital, London, UK

Stuart Taylor
Consultant Radiologist
Department of Radiology
Northwick Park and St Mark's Hospital
Harrow, Middlesex, UK

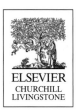

ELSEVIER
CHURCHILL
LIVINGSTONE

EDINBURGH   LONDON   NEW YORK   OXFORD   PHILADELPHIA   ST LOUIS   SYDNEY   TORONTO   2004

ELSEVIER
CHURCHILL
LIVINGSTONE

First published 2004

ISBN 0 443 07030 X

British Library Cataloguing in Publication Data
A catalogue record for this book is available from the British Library

Library of Congress Cataloging in Publication Data
A catalog record for this book is available from the Library of Congress

> **Notice**
> Medical knowledge is constantly changing. Standard safety precautions must be followed, but as new research and clinical experience broaden our knowledge, changes in treatment and drug therapy may become necessary or appropriate. Readers are advised to check the most current product information provided by the manufacturer of each drug to be administered to verify the recommended dose, the method and duration of administration, and contraindications. It is the responsibility of the practitioner, relying on experience and knowledge of the patient, to determine dosages and the best treatment for each individual patient. Neither the Publisher nor the editor assumes any liability for any injury and/or damage to persons or property arising from this publication.
>
> *The Publisher*

 ELSEVIER your source for books, journals and multimedia in the health sciences

www.elsevierhealth.com

The
publisher's
policy is to use
**paper manufactured
from sustainable forests**

Printed in China

Preface

More than the calf yearns to suck, does the cow yearn to suckle.

These wise words were used by Professor Samson Wright in the introduction to his *Textbook of Physiology*, which went through many editions, and they tell of the joy of teaching.

In a long career I have taught graduates and undergraduates at St. Pancras Hospital, the Hospital for Tropical Diseases, the National Dental Hospital, the London Foot Hospital, University College London Hospital, the Middlesex Hospital and, of course, the Royal National Orthopaedic Hospital. Teaching has been, to me, the source of the greatest delight and, therefore, when my name was given to the publishers Elsevier by undergraduates at University College London Hospital as a possible author of a textbook on radiology for undergraduates, it was a source of immense gratification.

It is, of course, impossible now for one radiologist to have a knowledge of all the diagnostic modalities in all the subspecialties, and I was glad, therefore, to be able to call upon the help and advice of colleagues in London, all of whom are acknowledged experts in their field. I would like also to add grateful thanks to Veronika Chambers, X-ray Film Librarian at the Institute of Orthopaedics UCL, for her editorial assistance. As editor, naturally I bear sole responsibility for the final product.

I hope future generations of medical students will enjoy reading this book as much as I would have enjoyed teaching them.

This book is dedicated to my daughter Nicola, the next generation.

London 2003 **P. R.**

Dedication

Dr. Peter Renton (1944–2003): a brief tribute

"Death cannot be and is not the end of life. Man transcends death in many altogether naturalistic fashions. He may be immortal biologically, through his children; in thought through the survival of his memory; in influence, by virtue of the continuance of his personality as a force among those who come after him; and ideally, through his identification with the timeless things of spirit.

When Judaism speaks of immortality it has in mind all these. But its primary meaning is that man contains something independent of the flesh and surviving it; his consciousness and moral capacity; his essential personality; a soul." *Milton Sternberg*

The above words could have been written with Peter Renton in mind. He will be remembered as a fine physician, a great and inspirational teacher, a devoted father and husband, and a true pillar of his community.

Aside from being a superb clinical radiologist, Peter's greatest gift, professionally, was as a teacher. He was equally at home teaching undergraduates and nurses as exchanging knowledge with specialist orthopaedic practitioners. Many medical students were pointed to a career in radiology by a chance encounter with Peter, and his tutorials for radiologists were renowned for their intellectual, practical and humorous content.

He loved teaching and he loved learning, and it is fitting that this book, his final text, is intended for the medical undergraduate.

Michael Rubens
London 2004

Contents

Musculoskeletal System

Imaging techniques 1: using ionizing radiation

Plain radiography

Formation of X-rays

A current is passed through the cathode in an evacuated glass tube. Electrons given off at the cathode pass to the anode. X-rays are formed. The 'number' of X-ray particles is proportional to the current passing through the cathode and to the time the current is on for. The 'energy' of the X-rays, which reflects their power of penetration through the body, is related to the potential difference between the cathode and the anode. An infant will require a smaller current (mA) and potential difference (kV), and less time (s) than a large adult.

Absorption of X-rays

X-rays are absorbed differently by tissues according to their density (Fig. 1A). Cortical bone, heavily calcified, absorbs all of the X-ray beam. The film beneath the bone, therefore, is unexposed and, when processed, remains translucent – appearing white on the illuminated X-ray viewing box. Air or gas (in the lungs or a joint) absorbs little X-radiation and so the underlying film is black (curiously described as *translucent* or *transradiant* in the lungs). Muscle absorbs fewer X-rays than bone, while fat looks nearly 'black' as it is of relatively low density (Fig. 1B).

Positioning of the patient

Plain films of bone are usually taken in two planes. The anteroposterior (AP) projection tells us that the X-ray beam enters the patient at the anterior surface of the body and exits posteriorly, where the film is situated.

Chest radiographs, however, are conventionally taken posteroanteriorly (PA). The part of the body nearest the film is the least magnified and better defined on film. On the chest X-ray, the cardiac width is best assessed when the heart, which is anteriorly situated in the thorax, is nearest the film, while a film of the thoracic spine is obtained in the AP projection, when the spine is placed near the film.

In most cases, the other projection used to image bone is the *lateral* view (Fig. 2). In some situations, such as the pelvis or shoulder, a true lateral view is unhelpful because there are too many overlapping structures. *Oblique* views are, therefore, used.

With *digital imaging*, the information acquired is stored on disk. Subsequent computer-generated reconstruction can take place in any plane. The radiation dose is also lower than with conventional radiography, as X-ray film is relatively insensitive to X-rays or light, while the computer-acquired image requires a lower X-ray dose for its generation.

Arthrography

Iodine-based contrast medium, alone or in conjunction with air, was used to coat the internal structures of a joint (Fig. 3). This technique was especially used to demonstrate meniscal lesions at the knee and tears of the rotator cuff in the shoulder. Since the advent of MRI, it is now rarely employed.

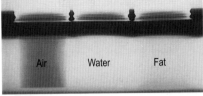

(A)

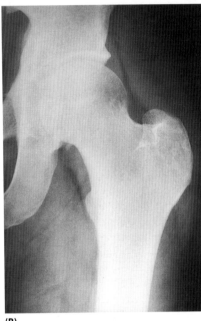

(B)

Fig. 1   (A) **Three specimen jars are placed in a water bath.** X-ray images have been obtained to show differences in radiolucency. (B) **Plain radiograph of normal hip.**

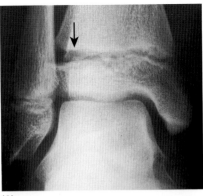

(A)

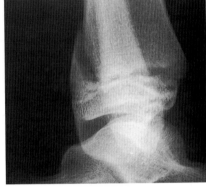

(B)

Fig. 2   **Fracture of tibia**: the need for images to be obtained in two planes. The anterior view radiograph (A) of the ankle shows a subtle abnormality – widening of the growth plate laterally (arrow). However, the lateral view (B) clearly shows posterior displacement of the growth plate, taking with it a large metaphyseal fragment (a Salter-Harris type II lesion). This is not visualized on the anterior view because the beam does not pass down the plane of the fracture.

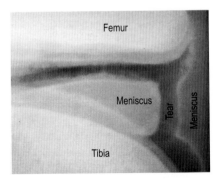

Fig. 3   **An arthrogram demonstrating a tear of the posterior horn of the medial meniscus.**

Myelography/ radiculography

Similarly, the injection of an iodine-based contrast medium into the theca was used to outline the spinal cord and nerve roots (see p. 14). MRI is now the preferred investigation to define disc protrusion and nerve root compression.

Radionuclide scanning

Isotopes, usually technetium 99^m-labelled methylene diphosphonate

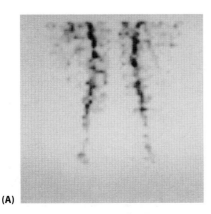

(A)

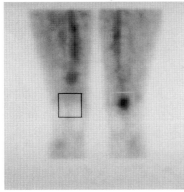

(B)

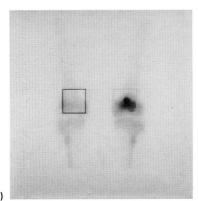

(C)

Fig. 4 **Radioisotope bone scan** showing an abnormality at the left distal femur. This was a localized tumour of bone, an osteoid osteoma. (A) The initial scan shows the isotope in the dynamic phase of the scan. The blood vessels are the site of tracer. (B) The blood pool image shows increased blood supply at the lesion. (C) The delayed image reflects metabolic activity at the site of pathology.

(MDP) for bone, are administered intravenously. Abnormal areas of bone show increased perfusion in the early or vascular phase of the bone scan due to local hyperaemia (Fig. 4). Delayed scans, usually obtained at 3 hours, show increased uptake of isotope by bone due to increased bone turnover at sites of pathology.

The technique is highly sensitive, often early on in disease, but non-specific.

Infection may be confirmed by the use of isotope-labelled white blood cells.

Computed tomography

Images are obtained axially, that is from top to bottom of the patient, in sequential slices – *tomography* (from the Greek *tome* – section, and *graphein* – to record). The X-ray source passes in a thin arc around the patient in earlier conventional and spiral scanners. The detectors move in a direction opposite to the tube in the arc. Modern multislice computed tomography (CT) scanners are more sophisticated, using up to eight active rows of detectors.

The attenuated X-ray beam, having passed through the patient, is then converted into images reconstructed by the computer. Computer acquisition allows accurate assessment of tissue density in Hounsfield Units (named after the inventor of the technique) (see p. 19) and reconstruction of images in any plane chosen by the operator. New technology allows rapid reconstruction of images in any plane (Fig. 5).

Vascular soft tissues have their images enhanced by the use of intravenous iodinated water-soluble contrast media.

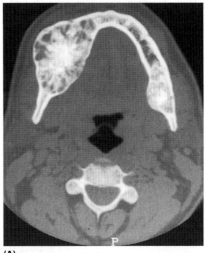

(A)

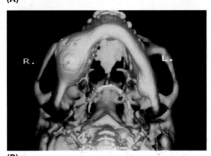

(B)

Fig. 5 **Fibrous dysplasia.** (A) CT examination of base of skull. (B) 3-D reconstruction. The expanding tumour-like lesion of the right side of the mandible is shown. The zygomatic arches are clearly seen.

Since the advent of MRI, this technique is less used.

For an up-to-date article on CT technology, see Garvey and Hanlon (2002).

References

Garvey CJ, Hanlon R. Computed tomography in clinical practice. British Medical Journal 2002; 324: 1077–1080.

Imaging techniques 1

Techniques used in musculoskeletal radiology
- Plain radiography
- Arthrography
- Computed tomography (CT)
- Radionuclide scanning, including DEXA (bone densitometry)
- Ultrasonography
- Magnetic resonance imaging (MRI)

Plain radiography
- Readily available
- Cheap
- Quickly processed
- Easily read
- Shows cortical bone well

Radionuclide scanning
- More sensitive, but less specific
- Gives accurate localization of disease
- Significant radiation dose

Computed tomography
- Demonstrates bone well but has a significant radiation dose
- Shows soft tissue also, but not as well as MRI
- Permits reconstruction in any plane.

Imaging techniques 2: not using ionizing radiation

All ionizing radiation is potentially harmful and, therefore, every effort must be made to diminish its use, even when necessary. Increasingly, alternative imaging techniques are being used that are assumed to be free of risk.

Ultrasonography

Diagnostic ultrasound uses high frequency sound waves (>20 000 cycles per second) that are inaudible to the human ear. A hand-held probe contains piezo-electric crystals that transmit and receive the sound waves. These bounce back at each tissue interface and the images of the received sound waves can be seen on a visual display unit (VDU) or stored.

Tissues of different structures have varying and characteristic echogenicity, and are thus separately identified. Pathology alters their internal structure and echogenicity on the VDU or film (Figs 1 & 2).

Magnetic resonance imaging

Magnetic resonance imaging (MRI) does not involve ionizing radiation, but instead utilizes the different distribution of hydrogen ions or protons in the various structures of the body and their different behaviour when subjected to high-strength, externally applied magnetic fields (Table 1). The field strength of the external magnets generally varies from 0.5 to 2.0 T (Tesla).

Hydrogen nuclei gyrate at frequencies in the range of radio waves or radio frequency (RF) and, under the influence of the magnetic field, their random orientation is aligned along the central axis of the magnetic field. RF stimulation deflects spinning protons and brings them into phase with each other. When the RF pulse is turned off, the system returns to normal. A measure of the time taken

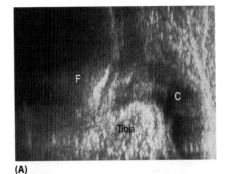

(A)

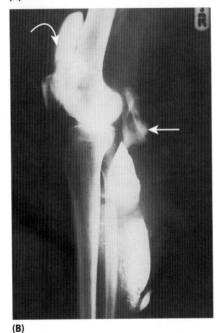

(B)

Fig. 1 **Baker's cyst.** (A) Ultrasound examination of the knee joint and calf. Internal derangement of the knee has resulted in an effusion and a posteriorly situated gastrocnemius-semimembranosus cyst. This is known as a Baker's cyst, after the surgeon who first described it. (B) The anatomy is clearly demonstrated after arthrography. Contrast medium has been injected into the knee joint. The distended suprapatellar pouch is shown (curved arrow), as well as the Baker's cyst (arrow), which has ruptured into the calf. This extensive rupture will produce pain and swelling of the calf and the symptoms resemble those of a deep vein thrombosis.
F = Femur; C = Cyst

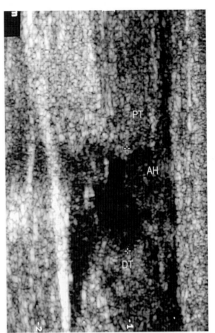

(A)

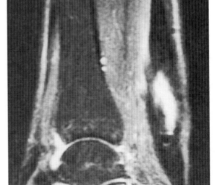

(B)

Fig. 2 **Tear of Achilles tendon.**
(A) Ultrasound. The tendon is of higher echogenicity (white), while the gap in the tendon, full of blood, is black. Courtesy of Dr P. O'Donnell. (B) A sagittal fat suppression magnetic resonance image of the ankle showing the tibia and bones of the hind foot. The tendo-Achillis is much thickened and shows extreme cystic and degenerative change centrally. The fluid nature of the cyst is well demonstrated (high signal) within the thickened tendon (low signal).
PT = Proximal end tendon
AH = Acute haematoma
DT = Distal end tendon

for dephasing to occur is the *T2* (transverse relaxation time), while the *T1* (longitudinal relation time) is that taken for the protons to re-establish their orientation relative to the external magnetic field.

Structures that have the highest concentration of protons – fat, fluid and medullary bone – have the highest signal, while those structures most deficient in fluid have the lowest signal (Fig. 3). Local increase in fluid due to

oedema, haemorrhage or inflammation, or malignancy, therefore, increases local signal, while infarction, cell death or soft-tissue calcification decrease local signal.

Table 1 **Magnetic resonance sequences in common use: signal intensities**			
	T1W	**T2W**	**Fat suppression**
Fat	Bright	Less bright	Low
Fluid	Intermediate	Bright	Bright

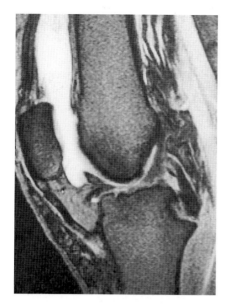

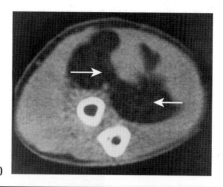

(A)

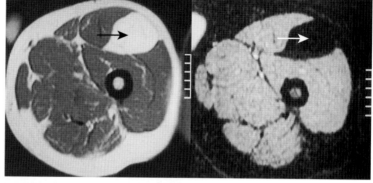

(B)

Fig. 3 **Joint effusion of the knee** – sagittal T2-weighted magnetic resonance image. There is a large effusion in the suprapatellar pouch (see also Fig. 1B). The quadriceps tendon and ligamentum patellae appear black, that is, of low signal because they are relatively fluid-deficient. Similarly, the anterior and posterior cruciate ligaments. The cortex shows lower signal than the bony medulla.

Fig. 5 **Lipoma** (A) A computed tomography scan through the forearm shows a large intramuscular lipoma, shown as a low attenuation (black) soft tissue mass (arrows). This is of the same attenuation as the subcutaneous fat. (B) **Septal lipoma** (arrow), (left). On the axial T1-weighted magnetic resonance image, its signal is identical to that of the subcutaneous fat; (right). On the fat suppression magnetic resonance sequences the fat is now uniformly suppressed and is black, as is the subcutaneous fat.

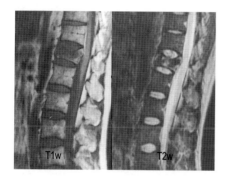

T1w   T2w

Fig. 4 **Burst fracture of T12** – sagittal magnetic resonance sequences. The vertebral body of T12 is collapsed. There is posterior retropulsion compressing the lower cord. On the T1-weighted image (left), marrow fat is replaced by low signal oedema, while on the T2-weighted image (right) the oedema is bright.

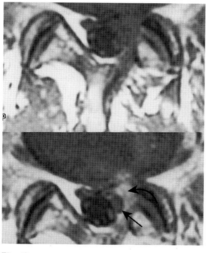

Fig. 6 **Enhancement of vascular granulation tissue around a nerve root after the injection of intravenous gadolinium** – axial T1-weighted magnetic resonance sequences. On the initial film (top) the root cannot be visualized, but on the later film, after injection, (bottom) the vascular nature of the soft tissues (curved arrow) around the emerging root (arrow) is shown.

MRI is becoming the investigation of choice for the musculoskeletal system, as both anatomy and pathophysiology are well demonstrated in any plane. MRI is not only more specific than isotope scanning, but is at least as sensitive.

In most cases *T1- and T2-weighted sequences* are used. T1-weighted images show better anatomic detail. Fat is bright and fluid grey. With T2-weighting, fat is grey and fluid bright. In both, cortical bone, tendons, ligaments and menisci are black (Fig. 4).

Fat suppression sequences cause the bright fat signal to be suppressed in the marrow and in subcutaneous and muscle fat. Muscle then appears homogeneously dark grey and the marrow black. Fluid remains bright and so any pathology with oedema,

infection, haemorrhage or hypervascularity clearly stands out against the low signal from surrounding soft tissues (Fig. 5).

Intravenous paramagnetic contrast media enhance vascular lesions when compared with unenhanced T1-weighted MR images (Fig. 6).

Imaging techniques 2

Uses of ultrasound in musculoskeletal disease
- Cheap
- Portable
- No ionizing radiation
- Demonstrates soft tissues well.

Magnetic resonance imaging
- Best imaging modality for soft tissues
- Demonstrates anatomy and pathophysiology in any plane
- Not as good for cortical bone as computed tomography, but excellent for bone marrow
- Very sensitive in the arthritides
- Costly, time consuming, not readily available.

Osteopenia 1: osteoporosis

Osteopenia, or loss of bone density – is a radiological appearance that has three main causes:

1. Osteoporosis
2. Rickets and osteomalacia
3. Hyperparathyroidism.

Osteopenia can be diagnosed on a radiograph as a visual loss of bone density, but is nowadays best assessed by DEXA scanning or computed tomography (CT) scanning, both of which use computers to measure attenuation of the X-ray beam by bone.

Dual energy X-ray absorption densitometry (DEXA scan)

X-ray sources of different energies are passed through bone and soft tissue in the area of interest – usually the hip, wrist and spine. The attenuation of the beam is assessed by computer. The results are expressed in terms of the number of standard deviations above or below the mean for an age-related control population (the 'Z' score) or with a young healthy adult population (the 'T' score) (Fig. 1).

Bone-density measurements at a site give a predilection for *local* fractures, while those obtained at the distal radius and calcaneus give a good prediction for fractures at any site.

Osteoporosis

Osteoporosis (Fig. 2) is responsible for much skeletal disease in patients over the age of 50 years because of the increased incidence of fractures. These occur mainly in the spine, proximal femur and distal radius (and ulna), as well as in the pelvis and upper humerus. The risk of these osteoporotic fractures is much higher in women. Thus, the risk of a femoral fracture is 40% in women over the age of 50, but only 13% in men.

Colles' fracture of the distal radius and ulna, usually caused by a fall onto an outstretched hand, increases in incidence in women between the ages of 40 and 65 years, after which the incidence remains constant; in males of all ages the (lower) incidence remains constant. There is a coincidental increase in the incidence

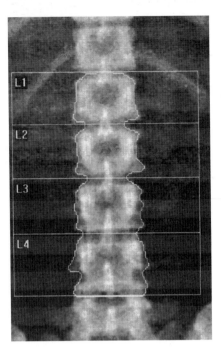

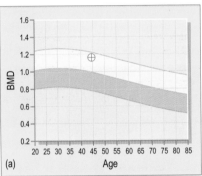

(a)

DXA Results Summary

Region	Area (cm²)	BMC (g)	BMD (g/cm²)	T-Score	PR (%)	Z-Score	AM (%)
L1	10.88	10.46	0.961	0.3	104	0.7	109
L2	11.66	13.12	1.126	0.9	110	1.3	115
L3	12.86	16.31	1.268	1.7	117	2.1	122
L4	16.38	20.28	1.238	1.1	111	1.6	116
Total	**51.78**	**60.17**	**1.162**	**1.0**	**111**	**1.5**	**116**

(A)

of falls in females between those ages. In the over-80s, perhaps because of an inability to break a fall with the wrist, a fracture of the hip is more likely (Fig. 3).

The incidence of femoral neck fractures is rising, not only because of an increase in the number of elderly (presumably osteoporotic) females, but also because of a change in lifestyles, with the elderly being increasingly more active. Fracture rates have been increasing, especially in women over 75 years, at a faster rate than the

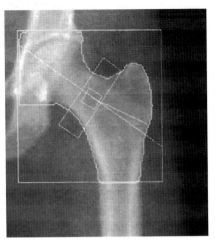

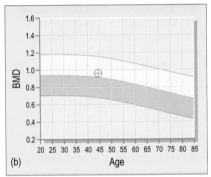

(b)

DXA Results Summary

Region	Area (cm²)	BMC (g)	BMD (g/cm²)	T-Score	PR (%)	Z-Score	AM (%)
Neck	4.61	3.85	0.835	−0.1	98	0.3	104
Troch	8.47	5.89	0.696	−0.1	99	0.1	102
Inter	12.58	14.60	1.161	0.4	106	0.5	108
Total	**25.66**	**24.35**	**0.949**	**0.1**	**101**	**0.3**	**104**
Ward's	1.04	0.80	0.774	0.3	105	1.2	122

(B)

Fig. 1 **DEXA scans for the lumbar spine and hip.** The patient scores above average, both in the spine (A) and in the femur (B). Ward's triangle lies in the neck of the femur between the major trabecular groups. It is the area within the small square. Lack of trabeculation in this region is often an early indication of osteoporosis on a plain film.

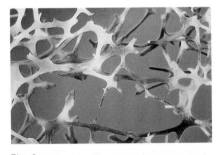

Fig. 2 **Osteoporosis** – 3D electron microscopic reconstruction to show structure. (Reproduced with permission from Gaw *et al. Clinical biochemistry: an illustrated colour text*, 2nd edn, Churchill Livingstone, Edinburgh, 2004.)

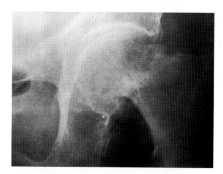

Fig. 3 **Transcervical fracture of the femur in osteoporotic bone.** Bone density is diminished.

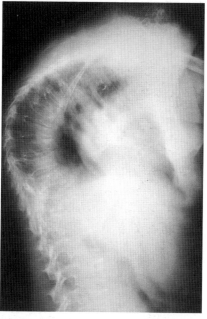

Fig. 4 **Dowager's hump** associated with multiple wedge compression fractures of the thoracic vertebrae. The bones are very osteoporotic. The vertebral cortices are thinned, but remain sharp and well-defined.

increase in the mean age of the population.

Women at risk for hip fractures include those whose mothers had fractures and those with any previously occurring fracture after 50 years of age. Most femoral neck fractures occur in winter and at home, so that icy surfaces are not necessarily involved. Their incidence is increasing; some 60 000 occur every year in England and Wales. In Finland in 1988 the incidence of hip fractures per 100 000 population was 174 in women and 78 in men. In that year, the costs of primary hospitalizations for hip fractures were US$66 m. In Belgium the mean annual incidence of hip fractures increased from 108 to 141 per 100 000 population between 1984 and 1996. Demographic changes accounted for only 10% of this rise. Up to 40% of these patients die within a year of fracture, often because of coincidental disease of the elderly.

Around 30% of patients at the age of 80 have fractures of vertebral bodies; these too are more common in women and are also increasing in incidence. Acute vertebral collapse causes back-pain localized to the area of the fracture. Subsequent fractures (these are unlikely to be solitary) are associated with even more frequent episodes of pain and, eventually, permanent discomfort. Vertebral deformity is associated with a scoliosis or kyphoscoliosis. A 'dowager's hump' may be present and clothes may no longer fit properly (Fig. 4).

The vertebral body fractures at its anterior surface and the upper end-plate becomes depressed or deformed. The disease is not necessarily seen in contiguous vertebrae – many may be uninvolved. Pain and vertebral collapse in the elderly may also occur with metastatic malignant disease, for example, from carcinoma of the breast. Metastatic disease often destroys the pedicle of the vertebral body, but osteoporosis does not.

Osteoporosis and resulting fractures are a complication of an excess of corticosteroids, either in Cushing's syndrome, or following excessive steroid administration (7 mg prednisolone daily seems to be the threshold dose).

Perhaps as expected, the changes are worse in post-menopausal females; however, they are also seen in children treated for juvenile idiopathic arthritis, which may be worsened by immobilization (see p. 25).

Radiological features of osteoporotic bone

Bone has a dense cortex and a relatively lucent medulla. After the menopause, cortical bone loss is of greater magnitude in women than is trabecular loss in the medulla. Excess endosteal resorption of cortical bone results in cortical thinning but, because the remaining cortical trabeculae are normally mineralized, the image of the cortex remains well-defined and sharp, though thinned. It stands out clearly in distinction to the medulla, which suffers trabecular loss and appears 'grey', while the cortex looks thin, pencilled and 'white' (Fig. 4).

Osteoporosis

Radiological appearances
- Cortical thinning
- Medullary trabecular resorption
- Fractures – wrist, hip, spine.

Features of osteoporosis
- Pathologically, the bone trabeculae are diminished in **quantity**, but are of normal **quality**
- Radiologically, the cortices are thinned but sharp, and medullary trabeculation is diminished.

Causes of osteoporosis
- Old age, especially in females
- Disuse
- Drugs – steroids, heparin
- Endocrine disorders – Cushing's syndrome, thyrotoxicosis
- Marrow infiltration – metastasis, myeloma.

Complications of osteoporosis
Fracture of:
- femoral neck
- wrist
- vertebral bodies.

These can result in deformity, e.g. of the spine (dowager's hump in the elderly female).

Osteopenia 2: rickets, osteomalacia and hyperparathyroidism

Rickets and osteomalacia

These are a less common form of osteopenia in the developed world. In the UK the cause is often dietary deficiency of vitamin D, especially in patients of Indian origin, combined with a lack of sunlight, which is needed to convert cholesterol in the skin to vitamin D precursors. In the USA the commonest cause is small bowel malabsorption, as vitamin D is fat soluble. Other causes may include kidney and liver disease.

Defective mineralization of osteoid leads to abnormal trabeculae, both histologically and radiologically. As the trabeculae are patchily mineralized, their image (or shadow) on a plain radiograph is not as sharp as in osteoporosis, but fuzzy and irregular. Trabeculae are ill defined in both cortex and medulla. Because of deficient mineralization, bone softening results, with deformities in both children and adults.

Rickets is the juvenile form of the disease, occurring before skeletal maturity and growth plate fusion. Children with rickets are weak and hypotonic (Fig. 1). Walking is delayed.

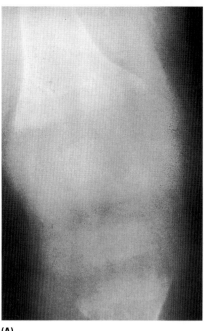

(A)

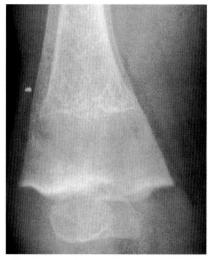

(B)

Fig. 2 (A) **Rickets.** Significantly diminished mineralization of the distal femoral and proximal tibial metaphyses and especially of the ossifying epiphyses is demonstrated. The ossification centres are barely visualized. The growth plates between the metaphyses and the epiphyses are broadened, the metaphyses are irregular and frayed, and the bone ends appear swollen. In the main, the epiphyses consist of non-mineralized cartilage. (B) **Healed rickets.** After treatment, the metaphysis has ossified and the growth plate is now of normal dimensions. The ossific nucleus of the epiphyses is well defined and mineralized. The image of the bone at the time of major vitamin D deficiency is shown within the area of bone remineralization following treatment (a 'bone within a bone' appearance).

Deformities of long bones occur and, in severe cases, of the skull base.

Radiologically, because of defective mineralization at the metaphysis, the growth plate is widened and irregular. Bone softening results in a broad metaphysis which, in the ribs, gives the beaded or 'ricketty rosary' appearance of the anterior ends. Joints appear swollen and deformed (Fig. 2).

Osteomalacia is the adult form. Patients present with bone and muscle pain with proximal muscle weakness, although histologically the muscles appear normal.

Vertebral compression due to bone softening results in back pain (Fig. 3).

The characteristic lesion, histologically and radiologically, is the *Looser's zone*, or pseudofracture. Looser's zones are seen radiologically as transverse bands of radiolucency surrounded by sclerosis (Fig. 4). They are composed of non-mineralized osteoid and are painful. Should they extend across the entire width of a bone, a true fracture results with considerable deformity. Bone softening also results in deformity, especially of long bones.

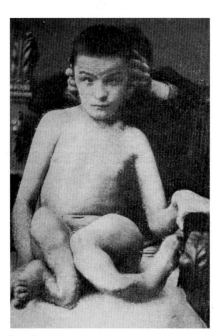

Fig. 1 **Rickets** – gross skeletal deformity. The patient has a myopathy and is unable to hold his head erect. (Illustration taken from Looser's book of 1920).

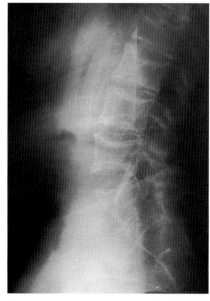

Fig. 3 **Osteomalacia of the lumbar spine.** The turgid discs cause end-plate depressions on the vertebral bodies. This is a so-called 'codfish' appearance.

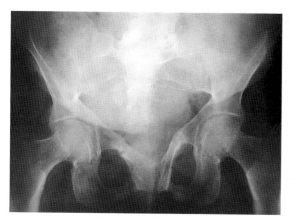

Fig. 4 **Osteomalacia of the pelvis to show Looser's zones.**
Transverse bands of radiolucency are demonstrated around the
obturator foramina, associated with skeletal deformity.

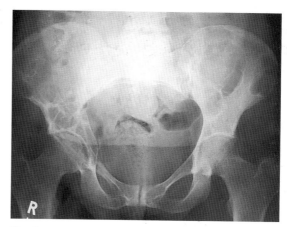

Fig. 6 **Hyperparathyroidism.** Multifocal areas of bone
destruction are demonstrated in the pelvis associated with cortical
thinning and expansion.

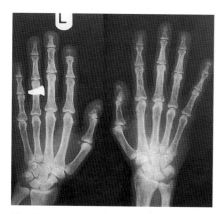

Fig. 5 **Hyperparathyroidism** – resorption of
the distal phalanges and of bony trabeculae
generally. The bones look ill defined.

chondrocalcinosis (but this is a
common finding in the elderly).

Osteoclastic stimulation also gives
focal areas of bone destruction –
osteoclastomas or *'brown' tumours* – so
called because of their macroscopic
colour, due to tissue necrosis (Fig. 6).

Focal areas of osteolysis in the skull
are often associated with reactive bone
sclerosis. An appearance likened to a
pepper-pot results (Fig. 7). Resorption
of bone around the teeth (the lamina
dura) also occurs.

Severe bone change is rarely seen
today as the chronically elevated PTH
levels are uncommon. Most patients
now are diagnosed early on routine
serum analysis.

Symptoms
Patient symptoms result from the
elevated serum calcium, giving the

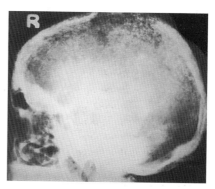

Fig. 7 **Hyperparathyroidism.** The
appearances are those of a pepper-pot skull.

classical '**stones** (renal), **bones**
(disease), **groans** (psychiatric
symptoms) and abdominal
overtones'.

In both adult and juvenile forms of
the disease, bone density is diminished
and both cortical and medullary bone
are ill defined.

Hyperparathyroidism

Hyperparathyroidism (HPT) is a rare
cause of diminution in bone density. It
results from an excess of parathyroid
hormone (PTH), usually caused by a
parathormone adenoma.

Osteoclast stimulation by PTH
causes bone resorption, especially in
the cortex of the bone. Radiologically,
Haversian canals – thin lucencies
containing cells – become more
prominent. Subperiosteal bone
resorption at phalanges is the
pathognomic change on a background
of osteopenia. Other changes include
distal tuft resorption in the hand
(Fig. 5). The elevated serum calcium
results in cartilage calcification –

Rickets, osteomalacia and hyperparathyroidism

Causes of rickets and osteomalacia
- In the UK, dietary deficiency of vitamin D,
  combined with a lack of sunlight
- In the USA small bowel malabsorption
- Also kidney and liver disease.

Rickets: radiological appearances
- Growth plate widening
- Metaphyseal cupping and broadening
- Bone detail fuzzy or ill defined
- Bone softening and deformity.

Complications of rickets and osteomalacia
- Fractures and deformity through softened
  bone
- Vertebral compression – codfish deformity.

Osteomalacia: radiological appearances
- Demineralization
- Looser's zones
- Bone softening and deformity.

**Hyperparathyroidism: radiological
appearances**
- Loss of bone density
- Subperiosteal bone resorption of the
  phalanges
- Phalangeal tuft resorption
- Chondrocalcinosis
- Brown tumours.

Osteosclerosis

In osteosclerosis the bones are increased in density. This change may be seen on plain films, on computed tomography (CT), and is generally associated with increased uptake on a radioisotope bone scan. DEXA and CT scanning quantifies the degree of change in bone mineralization, as it does in osteoporosis.

On a plain film, the bones appear 'whiter' than normal because they contain more calcium per unit volume. The extra mineral absorbs more X-rays and the film beneath such bone appears white, though the eye actually sees the brightness of the illuminated viewing box through translucent, unexposed and developed film. The image is the shadow of the overlying bone (see p. 2).

Increase in bone density often does not mean that the bones are stronger. Dense bones may be weaker because the crystalline structure of bone is altered and may fracture more often, just as does osteoporotic bone.

Osteosclerosis may be focal or general (Figs 1 & 2) and focal lesions may be solitary or multiple (Fig. 3).

General bone sclerosis is unusual in children and may be due to a sclerosing congenital dysplasia of bone, e.g. osteopetrosis (Fig. 4) (see also p. 28). This dysplasia of bone occurs in early (congenita) and late (tarda) forms. Often early cases have a more severe form of the disease. It may have a recessive form of inheritance. The affected patients may, therefore, not live long enough to pass the disease on. The bones are diffusely thickened and may suffer pathological fractures. When the marrow is obliterated by the sclerosing process, extramedullary haemopoiesis occurs with a large liver or spleen.

In the elderly patient, sclerotic lesions may also be solitary, multiple or general. Often the differential diagnosis is between Paget's disease (osteitis deformans) and sclerosing metastatic malignant disease, from the prostate in the male and breast in the female.

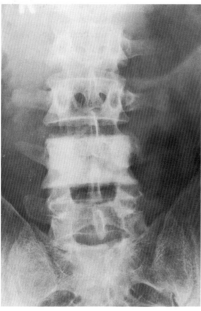

(A)

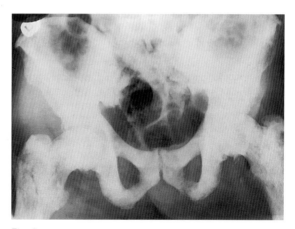

Fig. 2 **Metastases from carcinoma of the prostate.** A rather ill-defined but generalized osteosclerosis is shown. The sacrum, innominate bones and proximal femora are all generally involved. A few areas of normal bone density remain. Expansion of bone is not a prominent feature. In an elderly male patient, the diagnosis is that of carcinoma of the prostate.

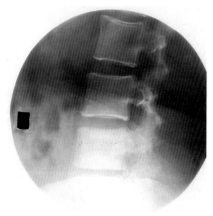

(B)

Fig. 1 **Paget's disease.** (A) Sclerosis of the body of L4 is an isolated phenomenon. The vertebral body is slightly enlarged in the transverse diameter compared to the vertebral body above. Cortico-medullary differentiation is lost. (B) The lateral view shows sclerosis of a vertebral body with new bone laid down anteriorly.

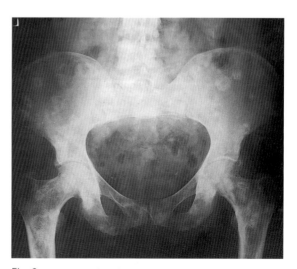

Fig. 3 **Metastases from carcinoma of the breast.** Multifocal areas of sclerosis are demonstrated in the pelvis, lower lumbar spine and proximal femora. They are tending to coalesce.

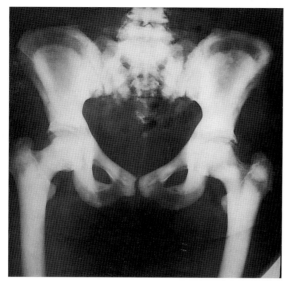

Fig. 4 **Osteopetrosis or marble bone disease in a young patient.** There is almost total and uniform increase in bony density. Slight bone expansion is also evident, especially around the obturator foramina. A 'bone within a bone' appearance is shown. This occurs because the disease is cyclical. Normal and abnormal bone are being formed intermittently and, in this patient, the abnormal bone is much more prominent than the few areas of normal bone.

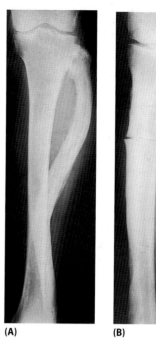

(A)   **(B)**

Fig. 6 **Paget's disease in long bones.** (A) The fibula is totally involved. It is thickened and, having overgrown, has bowed. It is fixed both superiorly and inferiorly. The bowing results from bone softening. (B) Sclerosis and expansion extends to the top of the tibia. A transverse pathological fracture is demonstrated. The deformity of the tibia has caused an oblique fracture of the fibula, which shows normal or diminished bone density.

Secondary malignant disease rarely expands the bone and may lie anywhere in the shaft of a long bone. Deformity follows pathological fracture through weakened bone, but bowing is unusual.

Increased density in bone is often associated with increased uptake on a radioisotope bone scan, for instance, in Paget's disease and metastatic disease, as these are areas of increased metabolic activity.

The CT scan shows increase in bony density and bone expansion, if present (Fig. 5). These images are generated using ionizing radiation.

At magnetic resonance (MR) imaging, an increase in bony density is seen as a loss of signal, as cortical

bone or dense bone contains much less fluid than does bone marrow.

Paget's disease of bone (osteitis deformans)

This is a disease of bone sclerosis and expansion occurring in the elderly. One, a few or many bones may be involved. Bone expansion and sclerosis is associated with softening and deformity (Fig. 6). The skull vault enlarges and the

cranial foramina are encroached upon, causing nerve palsies. Bone softening leads to transverse fractures. A hyperdynamic circulation with this vascular bone disease may lead to high output heart failure. Occasionally, malignant transformation to an osteosarcoma can occur.

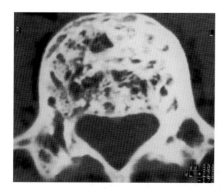

Fig. 5 **Paget's disease – computed tomography scan.** There is loss of normal cortico-medullary differentiation and overall the bone is expanded and shows a generalized increase in density. There are, however, focal areas of diminished density, or possibly normal density; vascular or fibrous tissue may lie within these areas.

Osteosclerosis

Osteopetrosis
- Occurs in early (congenita) and late (tarda) forms
- Early cases often more severe
- May have a recessive form of inheritance
- Bones are diffusely thickened and may suffer pathological fractures.

Paget's disease
- Causes sclerosis of bone with expansion
- Cortex is thickened
- In a long bone it starts at an articular surface and passes down the shaft in continuity
- Small bones are affected in their entirety
- The bone is softened and this causes bowing and deformity, as well as pathological fracture
- Malignant transformation to osteosarcoma can occur rarely.

Causes of focal sclerosis
- Paget's disease
- Bone infarcts
- Bone islands and other sclerosing lesions
- Chronic osteomyelitis
- Ossifying tumours, benign or malignant, and if malignant, primary or secondary.

Causes of generalized sclerosis
- Metastases
- Lymphoma
- Sickle-cell disease

(The above may be associated with splenomegaly. The bones are generally normal in shape.)

- Paget's disease
- Renal osteodystrophy
- Osteopetrosis and other sclerosing bone dysplasias.

(The above bones may be abnormal in shape.)

Painful back

Back and neck pain

Up to 85% of people in the Western world will suffer from back or neck pain at some time or other. This may be acute and relieved by analgesia, but may become chronic and result in severe disability, often with severe disruption of the patient's lifestyle.

The causes of back pain are many and may be found in all pathologies.

Causes of back pain

Congenital abnormalities
These may be secondary to spinal anomalies, with disc degeneration and nerve compression, for instance, above and below congenital vertebral fusions (Fig. 1) or scoliosis.

Infection
This may include simple, tuberculous or other rarer infections, such as brucellosis in endemic areas.

Spinal infection usually enters the vertebral body or disc by haematogenous seeding from a distant

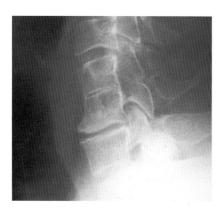

Fig. 1 **Congenital vertebral fusion** of C5 and C6 is demonstrated. The vertebral bodies are hypoplastic in the sagittal diameter. The facets are fused. The disc below is narrow.

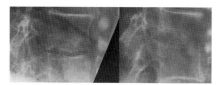

Fig. 3 **Spinal infection** – progressive destruction of the L1/2 disc over a month. There is loss of vertebral height, especially at L1 and the end-plates are progressively destroyed in association with discal narrowing and destruction by infection.

focus. The infection may spread from beneath the vertebral end-plate into the adjacent disc, which becomes resorbed (Fig. 2).

Radiologically, a mixture of cortical destruction and disc narrowing is seen. Further spread then involves the adjacent end-plate and vertebral body, so that two vertebral bodies and the intervening disc are involved in the destructive process (Fig. 3). Radionuclide bone scanning confirms the site of the lesions. Computed tomography and magnetic resonance imaging show local extraosseous soft-tissue change (Fig. 4).

Soft tissue abscesses around vertebro-discal infections are a feature of tuberculosis in the neck, thorax and abdomen. In the lumbar spine pus tracks into the adjacent musculature and a psoas abscess results, sometimes of very large proportions. The tuberculous process heals with extensive calcification, vertebral deformity and subsequent fusion. Fusion is more common with tuberculous infection.

Destruction of disc and bone may lead to cord compression and neurological deficit.

Trauma
This may range from minor spinal soft-tissue injuries, such as a 'whiplash'

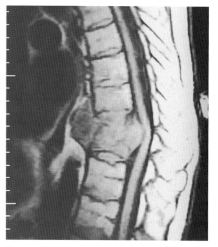

Fig. 4 **Tuberculous spondylitis.** On this magnetic resonance image at least two vertebral bodies are involved with an intervening disc. The disc is no longer visualised at the major focus of disease. A tuberculous abscess protrudes anteriorly and also posteriorly into the spinal canal.

lesion in the cervical spine caused by acceleration/deceleration forces applied to the neck, to vertebral compression following major trauma to the spine, such as a fall from a height or a road-traffic accident (Fig. 5).

Fractures of the spine may be *stable* and not subject to major deformity, or *unstable*, when the spinal cord may be traumatized, again resulting in neurological deficit.

Neoplasm
Benign tumours (see p. 18) can occur in the spine, often in the posterior elements, in children and adolescents. They rarely have serious consequences, though pain and deformity may result.

Primary malignant tumours of the spine are rare, but *secondary malignancy* is common over the age of 45–50. Malignant infiltration, vertebral and pedicle destruction and collapse cause unremitting severe pain and deformity, as well as cord compression and neurological deficit.

Metabolic disorders
Osteoporosis is commonly seen in the elderly and in the post-menopausal female. Minor inappropriate trauma may then cause vertebral compression, which is the cause of severe bone pain. These lesions are true pathological fractures.

Osteomalacia is less common but is also associated with vertebral collapse and bone and soft-tissue pain.

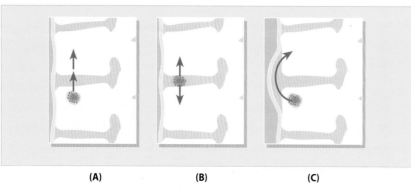

(A)   (B)   (C)

Fig. 2 **To show the spread of vertebro-discal infection.** The focus may spread from a vertebra into the adjacent disc (A), or from a disc into the adjacent bodies (B). Spread may also occur anteriorly beneath the anterior longitudinal ligament (C). This is common in tuberculosis.

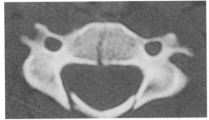

(A)

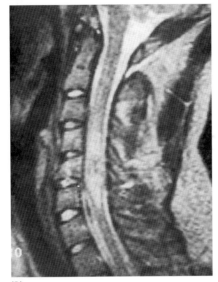

(B)

Fig. 5 **Fracture of cervical spine.** (A) The CT scan shows fractures of the vertebral body of C4 together with bilateral laminar fractures. (B) The sagittal T2-weighted MRI shows total disruption over a long segment of the cervical cord. The gap in the distracted cord is filled with CSF. Increased signal in the adjacent vertebral bodies indicate local haemorrhage and oedema.

Arthritides: rheumatoid arthritis, ankylosing spondylitis and allied connective-tissue disorders

Erosion of bone occurs in both rheumatoid arthritis and ankylosing spondylitis (see Box 1 for this and other commonly used terms). In *rheumatoid arthritis* in particular, the cervical spine is affected by erosive change involving the odontoid peg with rupture of the annular ligament, which may result in C1/2 instability and cord compression (Fig. 6).

Syndesmophyte formation

The erosions in ankylosing spondylitis heal with florid new bone formation (not a feature usually seen in rheumatoid arthritis) and spinal and sacroiliac fusion result. Vertically aligned new bone – *syndesmophytes* – fuses, giving a knobbly appearance, the so-called 'bamboo spine' (see p. 23).

Diseases of unknown origin

Paget's disease may also be associated with back pain, rarely because of malignant degeneration (see p. 10).

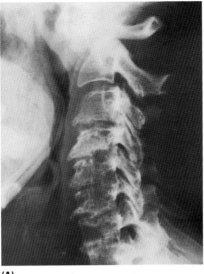

(A)

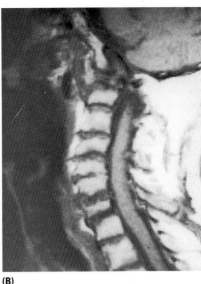

(B)

Fig. 6 **Rheumatoid arthritis.** (A) The lateral view shows forward subluxation of C1 upon C2. The odontoid peg is barely visualized. The space available for the cord behind C2 is much diminished. The soft tissues of the oropharynx are distorted. (B) The sagittal T1-weighted MR image shows compression of the cord, which is clearly seen below but not at or above the level of the lesion.

Box 1 *Terms in common use*

Spondylosis

It is probably incorrect to term degenerative disease of the spine *osteoarthritis*; this word is best used when referring to synovial joints. The term *spondylosis* (Greek: *sphondylos*, a vertebra – *osis*, a condition) is better used.

Spondylitis

As in *ankylosing spondylitis*, this refers to an inflammatory process of the spine.

Spondylolysis (Greek: *sphondylos*, a vertebra – *lysis*, a loosening)

Usually bilateral defects in the pars interarticularis separating the upper and lower articular facets of the vertebra.

This may result in ***spondylolisthesis*** (Greek: *oslithanein*, to slip). Usually L5 is displaced forward on that of S1. The intervening disc is often degenerate, while the posterior bony defects may be painful.

Osteophyte (Greek: *osteon*, a bone – *phyton*, a growth)

An outgrowth on a bone at an articular surface or vertebral end-plate, usually associated with degenerative disease.

Syndesmophyte (Greek: *syndesmos*, a ligament – *phyton*, a growth)

A vertically orientated bony bridge between two adjacent vertebral bodies, lying around the disc. Seen in ankylosing spondylitis.

Osteoarthritis (more correctly, osteoarthrosis) (Greek: *osteon*, a bone – *arthron*, a joint – *itis*, inflammation)

Chronic degeneration at a joint, usually age related.

Rheumatoid arthritis (Greek: *rheumatismos*, that which flows)

Painful back

Imaging of the painful back
- The basic and most commonly used investigation is the *plain film*, but this is not often diagnostic.
- With infection the *radioisotope bone scan* is much more sensitive than a plain film and magnetic resonance imaging (MRI) much more specific.
- Neurological complications may result from disc disease, infection, neoplasm or trauma. The cord is best imaged with MRI.

Disc disease

Imaging of the spine

In the UK 1.5 million patients undergo plain film radiography for low back pain, equivalent to 27 people per 1000 inhabitants. This is costly and also involves a significant amount of irradiation, especially if supplementary views are performed beyond the routine anteroposterior (AP) and lateral films.

The *plain film* is the cheapest and most readily available technique for investigating spinal disease, and is of value in excluding vertebral bone pathology and, by inference, disc pathology as shown by discal narrowing and osteophyte formation

(Fig. 1). The plain film also shows spinal alignment and changes at the posterior (facet) joints of osteoarthritis or rheumatoid arthritis, but is of little or no use in imaging muscles, ligaments, tendons or nerves.

In *radiculography,* a water-soluble iodine solution is injected into the thecal space (see p. 3). The contrast medium mixes with cerebrospinal fluid, which becomes opaque – white – to X-rays (Fig. 2). Discal bulging into the spinal canal compresses and distorts the theca and the local roots.

The side effects of radiculography include severe headache and, theoretically, meningitis. The technique also irradiates the patient. It has been largely superseded by MRI.

Computed tomography (CT) produces excellent images of bone in the axial plane and is good at showing

spondylolisthesis and canal stenosis. It also shows disc protrusion and local nerve compression (Fig. 3), but not as well as magnetic resonance imaging (MRI).

MRI is now the investigation of choice in the patient with low back pain (Fig. 4); indeed, there is a substantial case to be made out *against* the use of the plain film unless infection or malignancy is suspected. *Plain radiography* of the lumbar spine gives significant doses of irradiation to the patient, equivalent to 65 chest X-rays, while few examinations provide essential evidence for the diagnosis, prognosis or treatment of back pain.

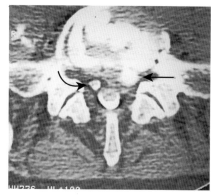

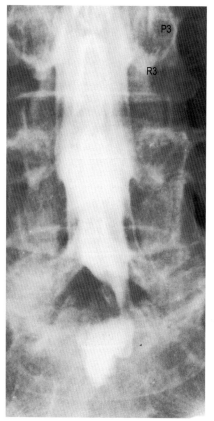

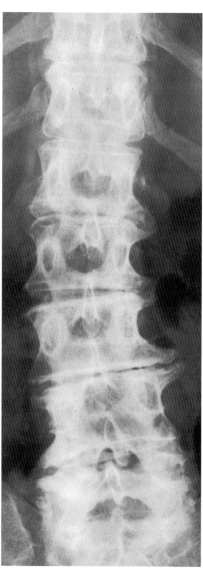

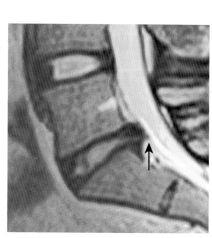

Fig. 1 **Degenerative change** is shown with discal narrowing, marginal osteophytic lipping and a degenerative scoliosis.

Fig. 2 **An anterior view of the spine at radiculography.** Opaque contrast medium fills the theca and outlines the contained nerve roots. The emerging nerve roots are contained within root sheaths. Each nerve root is labelled according to the pedicle beneath which it exits. Thus, the left 3rd root (R3) emerges beneath the left 3rd pedicle (P3).

Fig. 3 **Disc derangement – computed tomography.** The nucleus at L5/S1 level has been opacified by the injection of contrast medium (discography) and the theca has been similarly opacified (radiculography). On the left an opacified discal protrusion is demonstrated (arrow). The adjacent nerve root is not well seen but is present on the right (curved arrow).

Fig. 4 **Disc derangement – T2-weighted magnetic resonance sequence.** The L5/S1 disc is abnormal. It has lost signal and is less bright than the disc above, which is better hydrated. There is a large dorsal discal protrusion that indents the theca (arrow).

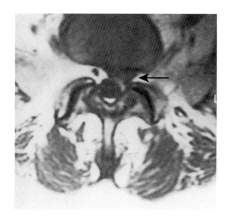

Fig. 5 **Disc derangement.** The axial T1-weighted magnetic resonance sequence shows a left-sided soft-tissue discal protrusion. The right nerve root is clearly seen as a low signal 'dot' surrounded by fat in the exit foramen, while on the left the emerging root is not seen. It is compressed by the discal protrusion (arrow).

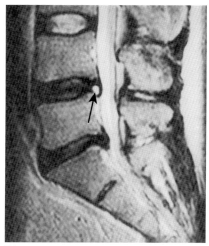

(A)

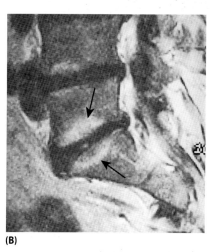

(B)

Fig. 6 **Degenerative disc disease.** (A) High intensity zone (HIZ). The L3/4 disc is of normal height and bright signal, but at L4/5 and L5/S1 there is loss of signal and dorsal discal protrusion. At L4/5 a posteriorly situated HIZ is demonstrated (arrow), indicative of a posterior annular tear. (B) T1-weighted MR sequence. Reactive changes in bone around degenerate discs (arrows) are often indicative of local inflammation and area associated with back pain.

Disc derangement

In the young adult, acute trauma to a disc may result in annular rupture and nuclear prolapse. The discal disruption is painful in itself, and the herniated discal material may compress the spinal cord and nerve roots.

In the older patient, disc degeneration inevitably accompanies ageing. The annulus fissures and its fibres separate. Dehydration reduces disc height. As a result, the facet alignment posteriorly alters, so that the local exit foramina become narrowed, leaving less room for the emerging roots. These become compressed – a process accentuated by new bone formation on the facet joints due to osteoarthritis (Fig. 5).

Disc degeneration is seen at MRI by loss of signal, indicating dehydration, and loss of height of the affected disc. Disc material protrudes into the canal. Tears in the annulus fill with fluid and are seen as *high intensity zones* (Fig. 6A). These are usually associated with pain.

Reactive change in the vertebral bodies around degenerate discs is also seen and is another indicator of a painful vertebro-discal complex (Fig. 6B).

Osteophyte formation
Discal narrowing and paradiscal soft-tissue redundancy are followed by the formation of new bone in these soft tissues – perhaps a buttressing phenomenon to prevent further deformity. This paradiscal new bone is usually horizontally inclined and is called an *osteophyte* (Fig. 1).

Disc disease

Acute back pain
(with or without sciatica but no serious infections)

Plain X-rays are not helpful except in the case of osteoporotic collapse.

Magnetic resonance imaging (MRI) should be considered after failure of conservative management.

Chronic back pain
(with no other evidence of infection or neoplasm)

Plain films are not sensitive. Many elderly patients have features of degeneration but are asymptomatic. May be of use in the young to exclude ankylosing spondylitis or spondylolisthesis.

MRI if surgery is contemplated.

Back pain with serious features
- In the young
- In the very elderly
- Neurological disturbance
- Generally unwell
- Previous malignancy
- HIV
- Weight loss.

Plain films may be misleading, but are usually performed. *MRI* is the investigation of choice. *Radionuclide bone scanning* is also of use to exclude metastases or infection. If MRI is unavailable, computed tomography (CT) should be performed over a limited area. Bone change is well demonstrated by CT scanning.

Infection of bones and joints

Septic arthritis

Bone and joint infection may arise through direct spread from a penetrating injury or by haematogenous spread from a distant source, such as a focus of skin sepsis.

In children, many infections of joints arise in the metaphysis, which is

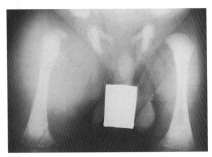

(A)

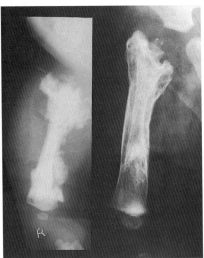

(B)   **(C)**

Fig. 1 **Septic arthritis.** (A) In a child the effusion may be of such a size that the hip dislocates. In this neonate the left hip is normally situated. The right thigh is grossly swollen and the proximal femur dislocated from the acetabulum by a large collection of pus within the joint. (B) Five days later extensive change is demonstrated along the femur. There is much periosteal new bone, especially proximally. Pus has spread down the medulla, broken through the cortex and elevated the periosteum, beneath which much new bone is laid down. (C) Three months later, after antibiotic therapy, the active pathological change has subsided and the appearances are those of chronic osteomyelitis. There is an involucrum with mature bone being laid down beneath the elevated periosteum, while linear sequestra are seen beneath the involucrum and represent the 'tombstones' of the previous cortex. There is extensive metaphyseal destruction. The distal femoral epiphysis is seen, and is growing, but it is likely that the proximal femoral epiphysis has been destroyed and growth proximally will be disturbed as a result.

intracapsular. This area is especially prone to infection as local blood vessels do not cross the growth plate, but terminate locally in large cavernous sinuses, where blood flow is sluggish, predisposing to the local deposition of septic emboli.

Pain, limitation of movement and systemic symptoms are presenting clinical features of septic arthritis.

Plain radiographs are of no benefit in the immediate phase of infection. Increased blood flow to the infected area causes osteoporosis, but this is not seen for 7–10 days. Up to 50% of local bone must be lost before demineralization is present on a radiograph. An effusion may, however, be seen (Fig. 1).

Late changes in septic arthritis follow bone and cartilage destruction with joint space narrowing and destruction of the articular cortex on both sides of the joint (Fig. 2); these can be assessed using plain radiography, computed tomography (CT) and magnetic resonance imaging (MRI).

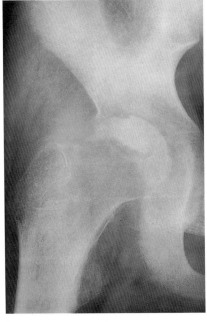

Fig. 2 **Septic arthritis.** Soft-tissue thickening is evident around the hip joint. The joint space is narrowed and the articular surfaces, especially at the acetabulum, are eroded. There is marked sclerosis of the femoral head. This is because it has been rendered ischaemic and necrotic, while the surrounding bone becomes osteopenic as a result of hyperaemia and bone destruction in infection.

Ultrasound enables the presence of an effusion to be confirmed and the joint is easily aspirated under ultrasound guidance (Fig. 3). Infection can be confirmed and appropriate treatment instituted.

Radionuclide bone scanning immediately confirms increased blood flow to the abnormal area and may show other abnormal foci due to sepsis elsewhere.

MRI shows an effusion and bone oedema, and is sensitive in the early diagnosis of septic arthritis.

Osteomyelitis

Once again, hyperaemia induces radiological osteopenia, which is not clearly seen on the plain film until some 50% of local bone has been resorbed. Bone destruction occurs, leaving a radiolucent cavity.

Bone destruction and necrosis

Devitalized areas of bone not resorbed by pus remain as *sequestra* (Fig. 4). These are linear strands of bone in an area of bone resorption. Sequestra are dense by comparison with vital bone. Devitalized bone, having no blood supply, remains dense.

Pus breaks through the bony cortex via a *cloaca* and elevates the periosteum. This lays down new bone

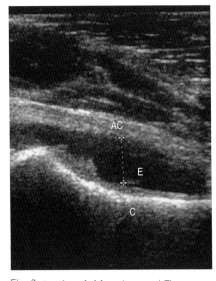

Fig. 3 **Septic arthritis** – ultrasound. The effusion separates the anterior capsule from the cortex of the femoral neck. (Courtesy of Dr P. O'Donnell)
AC = Anterior capsule
E = Effusion
C = cortex of femoral neck

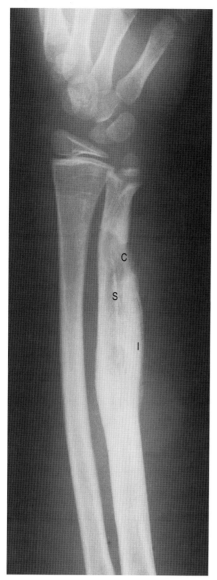

Fig. 4 **Osteomyelitis of the ulna.** Note the involucrum (I), sequestrum (S) and cloaca (C).

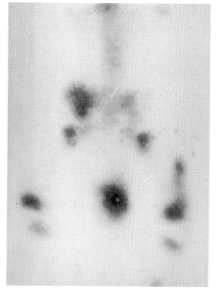

Fig. 5 **Osteomyelitis of the iliac blade.** The plain film had shown a destructive lesion and the radioisotope bone scan shows a significant local increase in uptake of the radionuclide. White cells can be labelled with an isotope; these cells migrate to the focus of infection and, after a lengthy interval, may be seen as an abnormal focus of increased uptake.

Table 1	**Bone infection**		
	Pain	Swelling	Osseous change
Acute	+++	+++	±
Subacute	+	+	+
			++
Chronic	±	±	++
			+++

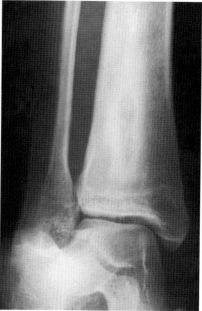

(A)

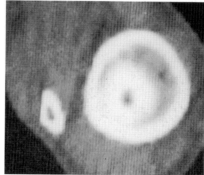

(B)

Fig. 6 **Brodie's abscess.** (A) The plain film shows a focus of destruction with much surrounding reactive bone change. (B) The computed tomography scan similarly shows a focus of destruction with surrounding sclerosis within the medulla.

external to the old, destroyed cortex (Fig. 4). Generally, such new bone is called a *periosteal reaction* or *periostitis*. In infections it is also called the *involucrum*.

As with septic arthritis, *plain film* changes occur late. *Radionuclide bone scanning* shows the effects of hyperaemia with increased blood flow to the affected area on immediate images, and increased uptake of isotope on delayed scans (Fig. 5).

MRI shows bone marrow oedema and fluid-filled cavities with increased signal on T2-weighted and fat suppression sequences, and diminished signal on T1-weighted images (see Fig. 4, p. 5). Cortical destruction and periostitis can be seen, together with sequestra. The local soft tissues are also oedematous. The anatomy is well displayed.

Chronic osteomyelitis may present as a bony defect with surrounding reactive sclerosis (see Table 1 for feature of acute, subacute and chronic infection). This is a so-called *Brodie's abscess* (Fig. 6).

Calcified tissues are always well seen at CT scanning, particularly the

involucrum and sequestra. CT shows chronic bone change in late disease, usually of marked reactive bone sclerosis and expansion.

Infection of bones and joints

Imaging of septic arthritis

■ Plain films are of no benefit in early disease

■ Radionuclide bone scanning is very sensitive early on

■ Ultrasound confirms effusion and allows aspiration for microbiology

■ Magnetic resonance imaging confirms disease in bone, joint and soft tissues.

Radiological features of bone infection

■ Destruction of bone

■ Sequestrum (pl. sequestra) – a portion of dead bone detached from healthy bone tissue (Latin: *sequestrare*, to lay aside)

■ Cloaca – a defect in the cortex (Latin: *cloaca*, a sewer)

■ Involucrum – the sheath of new bone that forms about a sequestrum (Latin: *involvere*, to roll up).

Localized bone lesions 1: benign tumours

Benign tumours in bone are in the main solitary, with some exceptions, such as multiple enchondromas or polyostotic fibrous dysplasia. On the whole, they tend to occur in younger patients during the periods of skeletal development (Table 1) and are surprisingly age and site specific. Because of their indolent nature, they are often seen as incidental findings or following a pathological fracture.

The radiological appearance of the tumour depends on its matrix or its cell type of origin (Box 1). Benign tumours arising in osteoid, fibrous or cartilaginous tissue usually mineralize, that is, show areas of increased density characteristic for the type of lesion, such as osteoma, fibrous dysplasia or an enchondroma (Fig. 1).

Lesions whose basic tissue has no propensity to mineralize remain radiolucent. These lesions include the simple bone cyst, aneurysmal bone cyst, giant-cell tumour and usually lipoma (Fig. 2).

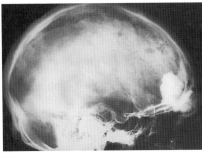

(A)

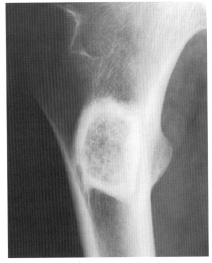

(B)

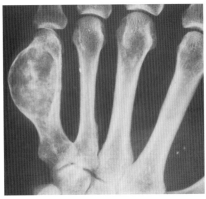

(C)

Fig. 1 (A) **Osteoma.** A large well-defined, very dense, sclerotic tumour is demonstrated within the frontal sinus. (B) **Fibrous dysplasia.** A characteristic site for this benign tumour of bone. The lesions may be slightly expansile and have a very dense margin. Matrix mineralization is indicated by hazy increased density ('ground glass'). (C) **Enchondroma.** Probably the most common tumour in the hand. It has a well-defined zone of transition between normal and abnormal bone and a thin rim of reactive sclerosis. Matrix mineralization is indicated by punctate calcification.

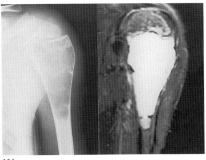

(A)

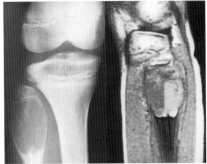

(B)

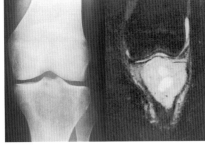

(C)

Fig. 2 (A) **Simple bone cyst.** The skeleton is immature. There is a slightly expansile lesion of the proximal humerus. It is unilocular with a few residual trabeculae. The fat suppression magnetic resonance (MR) sequence shows it to be fluid filled. (B) **Aneurysmal bone cyst.** Again, the skeleton is immature and there is an expansile cystic lesion thinning the cortex, but not here breaking through. The MR image shows fluid-fluid levels (the patient is examined supine). This is a characteristic feature of aneurysmal bone cyst and relates to the breakdown of blood products. (C) **Giant-cell tumour.** There is a lytic lesion of the proximal tibia. In this case, however, the patient is mature and the growth plates have fused. The lesion reaches the articular surface, a characteristic feature of giant-cell tumour. The fat suppression MR sequence shows the cellular nature of the lesion. It is not suppressed, unlike the marrow fat elsewhere.

Table 1 **Benign bone tumours: age of incidence**	
Benign lesion	**Age in years**
Eosinophilic granuloma	2–30
Simple bone cyst, non-ossifying fibroma, aneurysmal bone cyst	5–20
Osteochondroma (cartilage-capped exostosis)	5+
Enchondroma	10+
Fibrous dysplasia, osteoid osteoma	10–30
Giant-cell tumour	20–45

Box 1 *Characteristic radiological features of benign bone tumours*

Benign bone lesions are:

- well defined, with a narrow zone of transition between normal and abnormal bone
- surrounded by a band of dense bone of varying thickness, separating the tumour from normal bone
- slow growing, so there is little or no change on serial radiographs
- often round or ovoid until they reach the cortex, where their shape is altered. The cortex may become thinned and displaced so that the bone is expanded, but the cortex should not be broken through
- not usually associated with a soft-tissue mass.

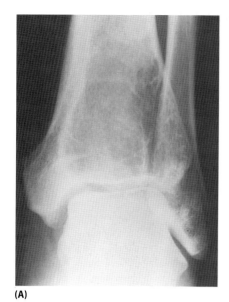

(A)

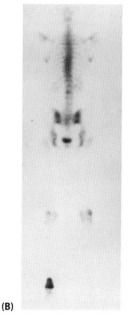

(B)

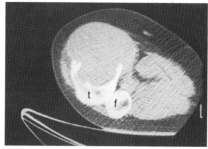

(C)

Fig. 3 **Giant-cell tumour.** (A) The anterior view radiograph shows an osteolytic lesion, which is slightly expansile, reaching the distal articular surface of the tibia. (B) The radioisotope bone scan shows this to be a solitary lesion. (C) The computed tomography scan shows a soft-tissue mass replacing the anterior aspect of the distal tibia in axial cross-section. The cortex is thinned, but preserved as a thin shell of high attenuation around the soft-tissue lesion. t, tibia; f, fibula.

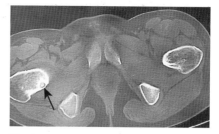

Fig. 4 **Osteoid osteoma** – computed tomography (CT) scan. The nidus (arrow), which is an actual tumour itself, is surrounded by reactive bone formation and, within it, ossification of the vascular osteoid tissue occurs. Calcific densities are white on the CT image, i.e. of high attenuation.

Calcifications, shown as white on the image, are of very high attenuation (Fig. 4).

Table 2 **Scale of attenuation: Hounsfield units**	
−1000	air
−30 to −100	fat
0 to 20	fluid
20 to 100	soft tissue
1000	bone

Computed tomography

Images obtained in the axial plane are computer reconstructed; the density of a lesion can thus be measured directly on the VDU. A lipoma has a very low density, or *attenuation* (from −30 to −100 Hounsfield Units (Table 2), in comparison with water, which has an attenuation of 0). Cystic lesions are of varying attenuation but still less than that of solid tumours (Fig. 3).

Magnetic resonance imaging

Here, the image obtained depends on the amount of water protons in the lesion but, as has been explained on page 4, images obtained at different weightings produce different appearances. Thus, while fluid is bright on T2-weighted and fat suppression sequences, the fat in a lipoma is suppressed (rendered black) on fat suppression magnetic resonance (MR) images. Cysts are bright (high signal) on T2-weighted sequences, while solid tumours have a signal similar to that shown by muscle (see p. 4). Calcifications have a low signal on all weightings.

The radiological features of benign lesions are altered by trauma, infection or secondary malignant transformation.

Radionuclide scanning

The radionuclide bone scan is strongly positive if the lesion is highly vascular and is avid for isotope, but if the tumour is fluid filled, only its periphery will enhance (Fig. 3).

Benign bone tumours

Radiological investigation
- Plain films
- Radioisotope bone scan to see if other lesions are present
- Magnetic resonance imaging (MRI) of the lesion to exclude soft tissue extension. MR examination spares the patient, who is often young, the relatively large dose of ionizing radiation from a computed tomography scan.

Localized bone lesions 2: primary malignant tumours

Tumours in bone may be solitary, or few, or multiple. Multiple lesions are usually due to metastasizing malignant lesions in bones or myeloma. Patients are usually over 45–50 years of age, that is, in the age group in which primary malignancy becomes common.

Age incidence

Primary malignant tumours of bone are usually solitary and occur in a younger age group than secondary malignant tumours or myeloma (Table 1).

Radiological features of malignancy in bone

Rapid growth results in poor definition of the lesion(s) with permeation through bone (Box 1 & Fig. 1). The cortex is rapidly broken through, especially with primary malignant tumours of bone, and a soft-tissue mass is formed, usually associated with marginal elevation of ossifying periosteum – the so-called *Codman's triangle*.

Table 1 **Malignant lesions of the bone: age of incidence**

Lesion	Age in years
Leukaemia, neuroblastoma	0–5
Ewing's sarcoma	5–25
Osteosarcoma	10–25, 60–80 (secondary to Paget's disease or irradiation)
Fibrosarcoma	20–40
Malignant lymphoma of bone	25–60
Chondrosarcoma	30–60
Secondary deposits and myeloma	45–80

Box 1 *Characteristic radiological features of malignant bone tumours*

Malignant lesions are:
- poorly defined, with a wide zone of transition between normal and abnormal bone
- without local reactive bone at the tumour–bone interface
- rapidly growing on serial radiographs
- seen to burst through the cortex and elevate the periosteum
- usually associated with a soft-tissue mass.

If the tumour has bone-forming potential, i.e. it arises in osteoid, fibrous or cartilaginous tissue, then the soft-tissue tumour mass will show irregular clumps of mineralization (Fig. 2).

Radioisotope bone scans are used to show the extent of the primary tumour,

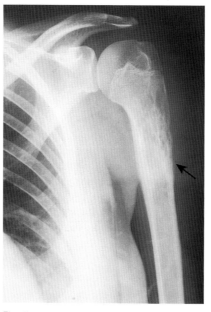

Fig. 1 **Ewing's sarcoma.** The proximal humerus is the site of an ill-defined permeative destructive lesion. The lateral cortex shows early destructive change and a marginal periostitis is also shown (arrow).

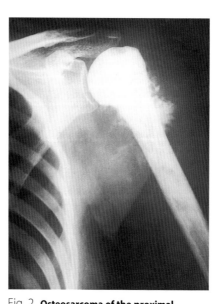

Fig. 2 **Osteosarcoma of the proximal humerus.** There is intense new bone formation in the proximal humerus with a large soft-tissue mass. Tumour new bone formation is evident in this. The appearances are those of a bone-forming malignant tumour.

but also to exclude metastatic lesions in the bones elsewhere and occasionally in the lungs (Fig. 3).

Computed tomography (CT) scanning is currently used to assess the presence of metastatic disease in the lungs or abdominal viscera. It is not now used to show the primary lesion. Magnetic resonance (MR) is the examination of choice, as it shows both bone and soft tissue.

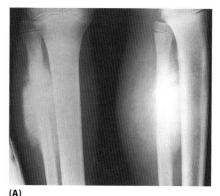

(A)

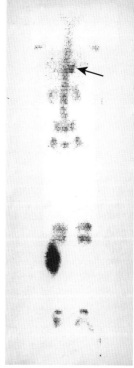

(B)

Fig. 3 **Osteosarcoma of the proximal fibula.** (A) The plain film shows a large soft-tissue mass with swelling of the calf. There is tumour new bone formation around the fibula. (B) The radioisotope bone scan shows added uptake of isotope by the tumour mass in the fibula, but also in the lung in a bone-forming secondary deposit (arrow).

At MR imaging, malignant lesions are often heterogeneous (Table 2 & Fig. 4), while benign lesions tend to homogeneity.

Metastases and myeloma

Metastatic lesions in bone are often multiple and may be small, without

Table 2 Signal changes of malignant lesions at magnetic resonance imaging			
Reason for heterogeneity of malignant lesion	**T1-weighting**	**T2-weighting**	**Fat suppression**
Pathological vascularity			
– arterial	low	low	low
– venous	intermediate	bright	bright
Cystic change	low	bright	bright
Necrosis	intermediate	bright	bright
Mineralization	low	low	low
Signal from basic stroma	intermediate	intermediate	intermediate/bright

significant bone expansion, with the exception of secondary tumours arising from the kidney or thyroid gland, or in myeloma.

Metastases should be investigated and demonstrated by a radionuclide bone scan of the whole skeleton (Fig. 5). Plain films can then be obtained of any abnormal areas.

Most secondary metastatic lesions in bone are destructive (Fig. 6), but some, usually from pelvic malignant tumours such as those originating in the prostate gland, cause reactive new bone formation and so are seen as areas of sclerosis or increased bone density, but without bone expansion. This feature distinguishes sclerotic

metastases from Paget's disease, which may also be widespread, but which is associated with bone sclerosis and *expansion.*

Myeloma deposits are very common in the spine, where they cause collapse but also expansion of bone (Fig. 7). This may result in cord compression. Characteristically, the pedicles are said to be spared in myeloma but involved with secondary metastatic disease.

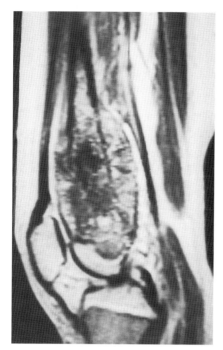

Fig. 4 Osteosarcoma of the distal femur – sagittal T1-weighted magnetic resonance image. The cortex is broken through. Tumour new bone is shown as clumps of irregular low signal material, both within the confines of the femur and also in the soft-tissue mass surrounding it. This corresponds to the foci of new bone seen on a plain film.

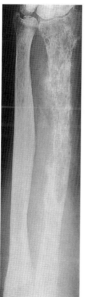

Fig. 6 Destructive, permeative metastatic disease from carcinoma of the breast.

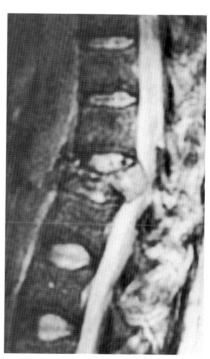

Fig. 7 Myeloma. The sagittal MR image shows the collapse with expansion into the spinal canal, causing it to be almost totally obliterated. Root compression results.

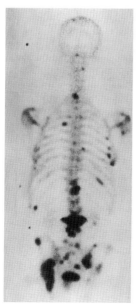

Fig. 5 Metastases from carcinoma of the prostate. A radioisotope bone scan showing widespread metastatic lesions.

Primary malignant tumours

Radiological investigation
- Plain radiographs – often requested by the GP for bone pain
- Radioisotope bone scanning – to show if any other lesions are present
- Computed tomography of the thorax – to show if there are intrathoracic metastatic lesions, which are often surgically resected
- Magnetic resonance imaging of the tumour – to show the extent of the tumour in bone and in soft tissue, and the involvement of neighbouring vital structures, i.e. nerves, arteries and veins.

Painful joint 1

Osteoarthritis (degenerative joint disease)

Destruction at joints is an almost inevitable concomitant of the ageing process, especially in those joints that are weight bearing, such as the hips and knees. Occasionally, premature osteoarthritis is the result of a congenital malformation of a joint, such as developmental dysplasia of the hip (see p. 26).

Some joints are rather more specialized structures than others. The knee and temporomandibular joints both have internal cartilaginous menisci, which are commonly damaged or become degenerate. The hip and shoulder joints are deepened at the acetabulum and glenoid respectively by a cartilaginous *labrum* (Latin: a lip), which increases stability.

In osteoarthritis, the initial process is one of cartilage loss in weight-bearing areas. This will be seen on a radiograph as narrowing of the joint space (Fig. 1). Subsequently, the subjacent bone is worn away at the weight-bearing areas, but new bone – osteophytes – often forms at joint margins. Bone density, especially in

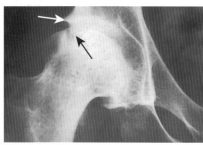

(A)

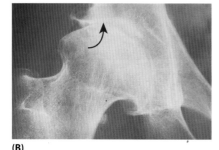

(B)

Fig. 1 **Osteoarthritis.** (A) Early osteoarthritic change is evident with a marginal osteophyte (arrow) and a cyst (white arrow). (B) Twenty years later, cartilage loss is evident superiorly, as shown by further narrowing of the superior joint space (curved arrow).

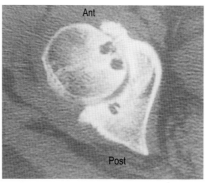

Ant

Post

Fig. 2 **Osteoarthritis.** The computed tomography scan demonstrates joint space narrowing at the hip anteriorly and, to a lesser extent, posteriorly. The articular surfaces of the acetabulum are irregular and some articular sclerosis is seen on both sides of the joint, a reparative phenomenon. The low attenuation areas are the result of cysts or geodes in the bone.

males, may be unchanged or even increased in areas of osteoarthritic change (Fig. 2).

Small cortical defects allow synovial fluid to be pumped into bone under pressure to form subarticular cysts – or *geodes* (Greek: *Ge*, earth; *eidos*, form, i.e. a sphere) (Fig. 2), which can reach a large size and undermine articular surfaces, which subsequently collapse.

Internal derangement of joints in osteoarthritis and following trauma

Plain films cannot show the internal structure of a joint. Joint space width relates to cartilage, and joint narrowing indicates cartilage loss. Effusions in joints can sometimes be seen on plain films by displacement of adjacent soft tissues, but internal structures, such as the menisci in the knee or the supraspinatus tendon above the shoulder joint capsule, cannot be identified. Previously, contrast medium would be injected into a joint – *arthrography* – and the internal structures shown with some accuracy.

Magnetic resonance (MR) imaging enables soft-tissue structures in and around joints, as well as the bone, to be visualized; bone oedema or bruising can also be seen. At the knee, effusions and bursitis can be demonstrated; the status of the menisci, cruciate and collateral ligaments can be assessed as well as the ligamentum patellae (Fig. 3). At the shoulder, the rotator

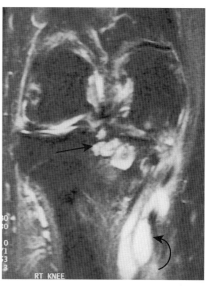

Fig. 3 **Osteoarthritis** – fat suppression magnetic resonance imaging sequence. The marrow is suppressed and appears of low signal, or black. Large cysts are seen in the proximal tibia (arrow). Note a subcutaneous soft tissue cyst (curved arrow).

cuff and other tendons, and the glenoid labrum are well demonstrated. At the wrist, the integrity of the triangular fibrocartilage can be shown, as well as the structures in the carpal tunnel. The ligaments and tendons around the ankle can now be seen. The tendo-Achillis in particular is well demonstrated on MR images (see Fig. 2B, p. 4).

Ultrasound is of use in showing structures outside of joints, but is of little value in determining the status of intra-articular structures, as bone does not allow the transmission of the ultrasound pulse. The ligaments and tendons around joints are well demonstrated.

Rheumatoid arthritis

Inflammatory changes in the synovium cause it to become hypertrophied and hyperaemic – *pannus*. The increased blood flow to a joint causes local osteoporosis, seen on the plain film. The hypertrophied synovium or pannus (Greek: *pannus*, a cloth) invades the underlying bone at the margin of the joint where, at that point, there is no covering of cartilage – the so-called 'bare area'. An *erosion* results. This is the characteristic lesion in rheumatoid arthritis. Cartilage erosion and destruction follows, with joint space narrowing and geode formation, and subsequent articular collapse.

The joints mainly involved, usually symmetrically, are the metatarsophalangeal and metacarpophalangeal joints, shoulders, hips and knees. Alignment deformities may result, especially at the hands. Secondary osteoarthritis is a late sequel of articular incongruity.

Imaging of rheumatoid arthritis

The *plain film* is the most commonly used mode of imaging in the arthritides. It is cheap, ubiquitously available and the images are easily read and interpreted. It has been shown, however, that early changes, especially in rheumatoid arthritis, are easily missed on plain films, that is, the plain film is relatively insensitive in the early stage of rheumatoid arthritis.

Early detection of erosions is important, as they do not heal in rheumatoid arthritis, and their presence early on in the disease suggests a poor prognosis and indicates the need for aggressive therapy (Fig. 4).

The *radionuclide bone scan* is a much more suitable indicator for the presence of disease, showing increased uptake early on – well before plain film changes are apparent. The bone scan is not specific, though the distribution of the abnormal areas on the scan can give a good indication of its cause.

The most sensitive and specific investigation is undoubtedly MRI. It is more sensitive in showing bone erosions earlier than any other modality and also shows the adjacent soft tissues, tendons, ligaments and joint effusions. The state of the articular cartilage is also easily assessed. However, MR examination of multiple joints is generally impractical because of constraints of time and cost.

Ankylosing spondylitis

This disease, which especially affects young adult males, is also an erosive arthritis. It is seronegative for rheumatoid arthritis, but HLA-B27 positive (Box 1).

Erosions commence initially on the lateral aspects of the sacroiliac joints and, subsequently, medially, and are inevitably bilateral. Further erosions develop in the spine at the vertebro-discal junctions.

Ankylosing spondylitis differs from rheumatoid arthritis in that the erosions heal with the proliferation of new bone, causing subsequent fusion (*ankylosis*) (Greek: *agkyloun*, to stiffen) of the sacroiliac joints. Syndesmophyte formation around the discs gives the so-called '*bamboo spine*' appearance. Eventually the spine is partially or almost totally fused (Fig. 5).

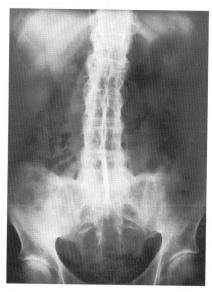

Fig. 5 **Ankylosing spondylitis.** There is bilateral sacroiliitis. Both sacroiliac joints have fused. A 'bamboo spine' is seen.

Box 1 Diseases of joints

Seropositive arthritides
- Rheumatoid arthritis
- Juvenile idiopathic arthritis (15% seropositive)

Seronegative arthritides
- Juvenile idiopathic arthritis (85% seronegative)
- Psoriasis
- Reiter's syndrome
- Ankylosing spondylitis
- Enteropathic spondylarthritides

Osteoarthritis

Septic arthritis

Gout

Haemophilia

Synovial tumours
- Benign – pigmented villonodular synovitis, synovial osteochondromatosis
- Malignant – malignant synovioma (synovial sarcoma).

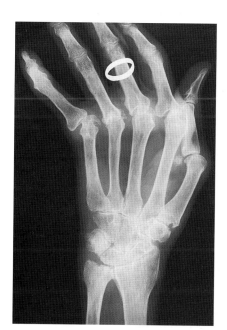

Fig. 4 **Late changes in rheumatoid arthritis.** Erosions are seen at the distal radius and ulna and throughout the carpus, and especially at the metacarpophalangeal joints. There is ulnar drift. Joint space narrowing is evident. In addition, there is widespread wasting of the soft tissues.

Painful joint 1

Radiological investigation of joint pain
- Plain films most commonly used
- Radioisotope bone scanning much more sensitive but non-specific, although distribution of lesions is an aid to diagnosis
- Computed tomography shows bone destruction well, but not usually performed in arthritides
- Magnetic resonance imaging is the investigation of choice, showing disease early in onset. Very sensitive and specific.

Painful joint 2: child

Osteochondritis

Fragmentation, sclerosis and collapse of bone can take place at various sites in the body. In some cases, the aetiology can only be surmised. These diseases are self-limiting, but the bone always heals to an abnormal shape, indicating in adult life that there was disease in childhood (Table 1).

In the femoral head, ischaemia may follow compression of the ligamentum teres by a hip joint effusion (see Perthes' disease, p. 27). The tibial tuberosity develops changes of osteochondritis at the site of traction by the ligamentum patellae (Fig. 1). The second metatarsal head develops osteochondritis (Freiberg's disease) because it takes the pressure of the foot – it is the longest metatarsal – when high heels are worn (Fig. 2).

The patients are all children and present with pain and swelling at the affected part; the underlying bone is fragmented and sclerotic. The local ligament, if there is one, is shown to be thickened on the plain film, at ultrasound and at magnetic resonance imaging (MRI).

Table 1	Common sites and causes of osteochondritis
Site	**Cause**
Femoral head (Perthes' disease)	Primary aseptic necrosis
Tarsal navicular (Köhler's disease)	? Primary aseptic necrosis
	? Necrosis following fracture
Metatarsal head (Freiberg's disease)	? Primary aseptic necrosis
	? Necrosis following fracture
Lunate (Kienböck's disease)	? Primary aseptic necrosis
	? Necrosis following fracture
Tibial tubercle (Osgood-Schlatter disease)	Necrosis following partial avulsion of patellar tendon
Lower pole of patella (Sinding-Larsen disease)	Necrosis following partial avulsion of patellar tendon
Vertebral body (Calvé's disease)	Eosinophilic granuloma
(Adapted from Catto M. *Aseptic necrosis of bone*. Excerpta Medica, Amsterdam, 1976 with kind permission)	

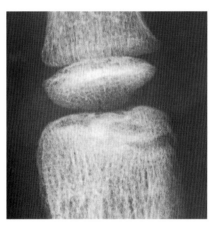

Fig. 2 **Freiberg's disease.**

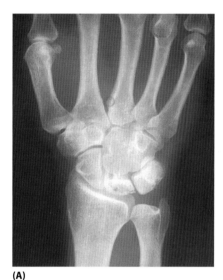

(A)

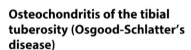

Fig. 1 **Osgood-Schlatter's disease.**
Irregularity of the tibial tuberosity is associated with thickening of the overlying soft tissues at the insertion of the ligamentum patellae. This is always swollen, and painful on palpation.

Osteochondritis of the tibial tuberosity (Osgood-Schlatter's disease)

This is a common cause of a painful knee in a child. The tibial tuberosity must always be inspected in such cases. The overlying soft tissues are always thickened – this change is an essential part of the diagnosis. The ligamentum patellae is also thickened and oedematous. Radiologically, the tuberosity becomes irregular, fragmented and sclerotic (Fig. 1).

In adult life, previous disease is shown by residual fragmentation of the tibial tuberosity.

Kienböck's disease

Avascular necrosis of the lunate may well be post-traumatic. This bone becomes fragmented and sclerotic (Fig. 3).

Osteochondritis dissecans

This is another cause of painful joints, especially at the knee in adolescents. A

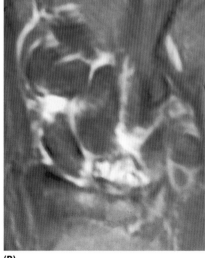

(B)

Fig. 3 **Kienböck's disease.** (A) The plain film shows collapse and sclerosis of this bone. The sclerosis indicates bone death. (B) Coronal fat suppression MR sequence of the wrist in another patient shows the necrotic lunate to be very oedematous. The fluid stands out clearly on the fat suppressed image.

defect is seen, most commonly at the medial femoral condyle, less commonly at the lateral, and occasionally bilaterally. There may be a family history of this disease.

The defect is often well corticated and contains the fragment of bone that has become dissected or separated off. Occasionally, this fragment comes to lie loose within the joint space, where it may grow, causing locking.

Radiologically, the lesion is well shown with plain films, as it relates largely to cortical bone (Fig. 4). MRI demonstrates the dissected fragment usually lying in the condylar defect and shows whether the overlying

articular cartilage is intact. There may be overlying bone oedema.

Other causes of joint pain in children

Juvenile idiopathic arthritis

Juvenile idiopathic arthritis (JIA) presents with a painful joint or joints; one or many may be involved (Fig. 5). The affected joints will initially be swollen, red, hot and painful. Subsequent hyperaemia results in overgrowth of bone with advancement of the skeletal maturity, as shown by more rapid ossification of the ossification centres in affected joints. The ossification centres, however, have an abnormal, rather angular configuration (Fig. 6).

Erosions are not an early feature in this disease. Only 15% of children with

JIA are seropositive and only these tend to have an erosive arthritis.

Plain radiography shows the disease in its earliest phase; soft tissue swelling and bone overgrowth occur. Serial films show progression of the disease.

Radionuclide scanning may be useful in confirming activity and showing if other joints are involved. This may be clinically apparent, however.

MRI will confirm the presence of an effusion and of bone oedema, as well as overgrowth of the affected ossification centres.

Because hyperaemia results in accelerated maturity of the bones around a joint, growth plate fusion takes place earlier than it would otherwise, and the affected limb, or part of a limb, ends up smaller than normal despite initial overgrowth.

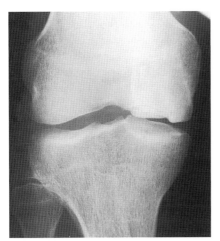

(A)

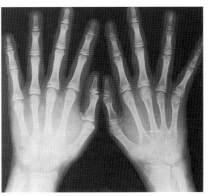

Fig. 5 **Juvenile idiopathic arthritis.** The left hand in this child is normal but on the right there is muscle wasting, osteoporosis and abnormal modelling of the carpal bones. These are overgrown with narrow joint spaces. Synovitis and hyperaemia cause these changes.

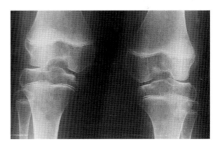

Fig. 6 **Juvenile idiopathic arthritis.** Both knees are affected in this child. There is marked osteoporosis. The epiphyses are ossified in advance of the chronological age of the patient. They have an abnormal contour, being overgrown.

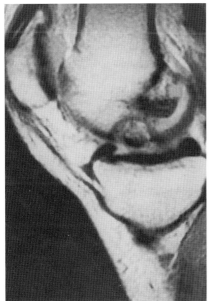

(B)

Fig. 4 **Osteochondritis dissecans.** (A) The plain film shows a large defect at the medial femoral condyle which is occupied by a well-defined ossicle. (B) In another patient the MR image shows the low signal ossicle lying within a defect of the medial femoral condyle, surrounded by fluid.

Painful joint 2: child

Sites of osteochondritis dissecans
- Knee
- Talus
- Capitellum
- Humeral head.

Radiological investigation of a painful joint in a child
- Initial radiological investigation is usually the *plain film*. This is cheap, readily available and easy to interpret.
- The local soft tissues must be inspected as well as the underlying bone. Soft tissue swelling may be present.
- A painful joint with a negative X-ray may require a *radioisotope scan* or *MRI examination*, both of which are much more sensitive in the detection of joint abnormalities than the plain film.

Abnormal hip in childhood

Infant hip

Developmental dysplasia of the hip

The acetabular roof at birth is largely cartilaginous superiorly, but nevertheless contains and covers the femoral head; it subsequently ossifies. If this cartilage is defective, subsequent ossification leads to a sloping, as opposed to a horizontal, acetabular roof, thus allowing the femoral head to sublux laterally or dislocate (Fig. 1). Developmental dysplasia of the hip (DDH) is more common in females and may be familial. It is more common after breech presentations.

At *ultrasound* the lateral bony acetabular rim, the cartilaginous labrum, the triradiate cartilage and the cartilaginous femoral head are all identified, and their relationships can be assessed, both statically and dynamically (Fig. 2).

The *plain film* is no longer routinely used in determining the presence of developmental dysplasia of the hip in the neonate. However, in the older child, it is used to assess progress of the dysplasia, both before and after surgery, that is, when more of the epiphyseal and acetabular cartilage is ossified. The shallow acetabulum is seen, as is the displaced proximal femoral capital epiphysis. A false acetabulum may be visualised. Shenton's line is broken by the upward subluxation of the femur (Fig. 1).

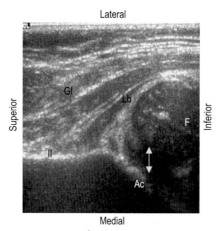

Fig. 2 **Developmental dysplasia of the hip** – ultrasound. Coronal scan. Note the shallow acetabulum (Ac), which covers only one-third of the femoral head, and displacement of the femoral head (F) laterally. Il, ilium; Gl, gluteal muscle; Lb, labrum. (Courtesy of Dr R. Green)

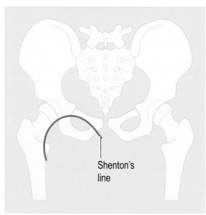

(A)

(B)

Fig. 1 (A) **Bilateral developmental dysplasia of the hip.** The child is around 6 months of age. The acetabula are sloping and dysplastic. The femoral heads are laterally subluxed. Shenton's line is discontinuous. (B) Diagram to show position of Shenton's line.

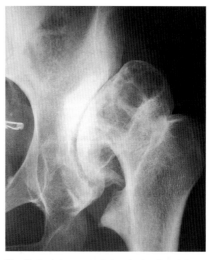

Fig. 3 **Developmental dysplasia of the hip – late effects.** This film, taken in adult life, shows the unreduced femoral head and the dysplastic and sloping acetabular roof. There is much new bone medially within the acetabulum, as it has never had the pressure of a normal femoral head upon it. Secondary osteoarthritic changes are evident, with narrowing of the joint space and reactive sclerosis around the dysplastic hip joint.

In the untreated case, the femoral head is laterally subluxed within a shallow acetabulum. It is flattened. Secondary degenerative changes supervene (Fig. 3).

Hip at 6–8 years

Aside from septic arthritis, which may present at any time, children presenting with a painful hip at 6–8 years should have an irritable hip and Perthes' disease excluded.

Irritable hip syndrome

The child complains of pain and limitation of movement, similar perhaps to the symptoms of septic arthritis (see p. 16). The plain film may show widening of the hip joint space due to an effusion, which should be measured and compared with the normal side (Fig. 4).

Ultrasound allows the joint width to be accurately measured and subsequent aspiration of the joint; infection can thus be excluded (Fig. 5).

Should pain persist, a radionuclide bone scan may show diminished or no perfusion in the femoral head (Fig. 6). Magnetic resonance imaging (MRI) also shows the effusion and signal changes in the femoral head.

Perthes' disease

On the *plain film*, with established Perthes' disease (Box 1) (see also p. 24), the devitalized ossific nucleus in the femoral capital epiphysis, that is, the mineralized part, collapses and appears sclerotic, fragmented and fissured (Fig. 7).

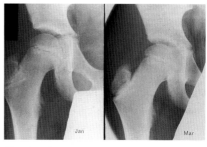

Fig. 4 **Irritable hip syndrome.** Some widening of the right hip joint, seen in January, has reverted to a normal appearance in March. The effusion has resolved.

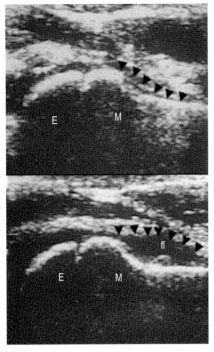

Fig. 5 **Irritable hip syndrome.** Sagittal ultrasound scan of child's hip. In the upper and lower image the high echogenicity of the cortical bone of the epiphysis (E) and metaphysis (M) is noted. The arrowheads indicate the joint capsule; in the upper image this is concave along the femoral neck but in the lower image is convex to the femoral neck beneath which there is anechoic fluid (fl). (Courtesy of Dr R. Green)

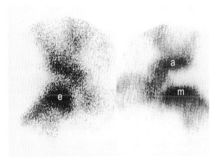

Fig. 6 **Perthes' disease – radioisotope bone scan.** There is a large area of photopenia, or defect of isotope, on the left between the acetabular roof (a) and the metaphysis of the femoral neck (m). On the right the epiphysis (e) is the site of considerable uptake of isotope.

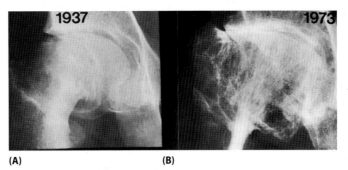

(A)   **(B)**

Fig. 9 **Slipped epiphysis.** (A) The femoral head no longer sits on the neck, but has slipped inferomedially. (B) After many years the patient has developed severe secondary osteoarthritis.

MR imaging is of great value in assessing the vascularity, or lack of it, in the femoral head, as well as subsequent repair (Fig. 8).

Box 1 *Irritable hip syndrome/Perthes' disease*

Initial phase
- Plain film – are the bony structures normal?
- Radioisotope bone scan – shows a 'cold' or photopenic area at the site of decreased perfusion
- Ultrasound shows the effusion and allows aspiration
- Magnetic resonance imaging shows the effusion and oedema of the femoral head.

Later phase
- Plain film: bony change is well seen. Follow-up to show healing on serial films
- Magnetic resonance imaging will also show the extent of the necrotic segment.

Healing inevitably occurs, but never to a normal round femoral head and congruous acetabulum. Perthes' disease ends with a flattened, mushroom-shaped femoral head. Secondary osteoarthritis supervenes many years later.

Adolescent hip

Slipped femoral capital epiphysis
This is a cause of hip pain around puberty. A stress fracture occurs through the growth plate and the femoral head slips inferomedially (Fig. 9). It may need to be reduced and pinned.

The slip is seen on anteroposterior (AP) and oblique plain films. Computed tomography (CT) demonstrates the changes well, but the gonad radiation dose is high.

Secondary osteoarthritis due to articular incongruity results early in adult life.

Septic arthritis
See page 16.

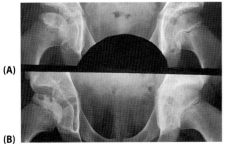

(A)

(B)

Fig. 7 **Perthes' disease – early and late.** (A) The initial radiograph shows early collapse of the right femoral head. The cortex superiorly is no longer continuous. (B) The later radiograph shows established disease. The femoral head is flattened, sclerotic and fissured.

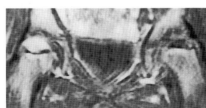

Fig. 8 **Perthes' disease.** Coronal T1-weighted MR sequence showing a normal right femoral head, with fat in the marrow of the femoral head. On the left there is a signal void. The low signal in the femoral head indicates necrosis and collapse, and would be seen as sclerosis on a radiograph.

Abnormal hip in childhood

Causes of the abnormal hip in childhood
- *Infancy* – developmental dysplasia of the hip
- *Child aged between 6 and 8 years* – Perthes' disease
- *Puberty* – slipped femoral capital epiphysis
- *All ages* – juvenile idiopathic arthritis.

Congenital disorders and non-accidental injury

Dysplasias (Greek: *dys*, bad; *plasia*, forming)

Plain films of multiple bones and joints are usually diagnostic. Further imaging is not usually necessary.

Achondroplasia

Probably the commonest skeletal dysplasia, achondroplasia is characterized by marked dwarfism due especially to limb shortening. The hands too are short and stubby – the *trident hand* – as the metacarpals are all of the same length (Fig. 1). The spinal canal is much narrowed as the pedicles are short and the space between them diminishes inferiorly in the lumbar spine (in the normal spine the interpedicular distance increases inferiorly) (Fig. 2). Severe canal stenosis with nerve compression results. There is a lumbar hyperlordosis, giving prominent buttocks, and a large calvarium with depressed nasal bones.

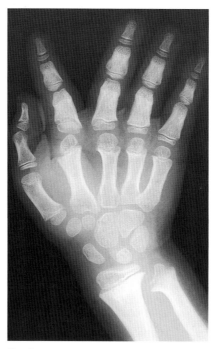

Fig. 1 **Achondroplasia – 'trident' hand.** Short metacarpals and short stubby phalanges. The fingers are of the same length.

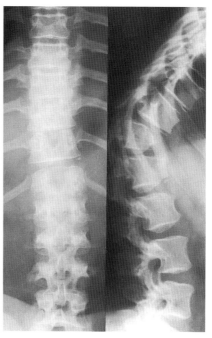

Fig. 2 **Achondroplasia.** Narrowing of the interpedicular distances inferiorly and short pedicles cause canal stenosis in the lumbar spine. There is scalloping of the posterior aspects of the vertebral bodies. Instability also gives deformity at the thoracolumbar junction.

Osteopetrosis (marble bones)

This is a sclerosing bone dysplasia in which bones are uniformly or intermittently of increased density, and also broadened (see also p. 10) – another cause of the *Erlenmeyer flask* appearance.

Medullary obliteration by dense bone may result in anaemia. Extramedullary haemopoiesis then occurs.

As the skull vault thickens, the foramina become encroached upon. Nerve palsies and blindness occur in severely affected cases.

Although denser, the bones suffer fractures, but cannot, however, be confused with osteogenesis imperfecta (see below), where the bones are usually osteoporotic.

Neurofibromatosis

This dysplasia has multiple features. Skin changes include six or more café-au-lait spots and multiple neural skin tumours.

Overgrowth of a limb or part of a limb also occurs. Both bone and soft tissues can be involved. The enlarged limb is often supplied by a plexiform neurofibroma.

Some bone lesions are dysplastic in origin. Resorption of the tibia at its distal midshaft is followed by a pathological fracture that does not heal and at which the bone ends resorb, giving a *pseudarthrosis* with local deformity (Fig. 3).

Occasionally, the sphenoid bone does not develop and the bony orbit is defective posteriorly (the *empty orbit*). CSF pulsation causes pulsating exophthalmos.

Other changes in bone, such as rib notching, may be caused by the presence of neural tumours on the intercostal nerves, which erode bone. Tumours on spinal nerves may cause enlargement of the intervertebral exit foramina. Vertebral defects also occur, with anterior and posterior scalloping of vertebral bodies.

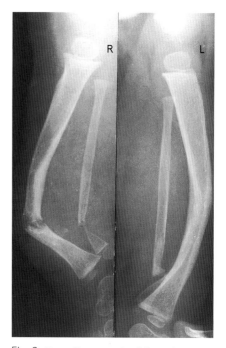

Fig. 3 **Neurofibromatosis – bilateral pseudarthroses.** The bowing deformity becomes progressive and results in fractures.

Osteogenesis imperfecta

This is a congenital dysplasia of bone occurring in a variety of forms of differing severity. A simple classification, of a severe recessive form and a milder, dominant form has been superseded by a more complicated classification with four basic types with further subtypes. Changes are often

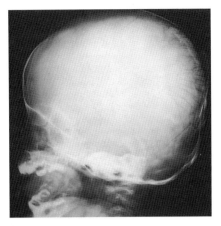

Fig. 4 **Osteogenesis imperfecta.** Delayed ossification and mineralisation of the sutures, within which lie numerous sutural or Wormian bones.

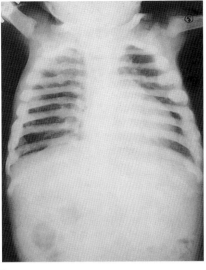

Fig. 6 **Non-accidental injury.** Healing rib fractures are shown, both posteriorly and laterally, as areas of bone expansion.

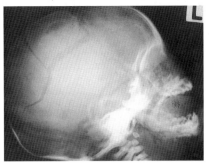

Fig. 7 **Non-accidental injury.** The wide lucencies in the parietal region should not be thought of as normal variants or sutures. The margins are too straight and well defined.

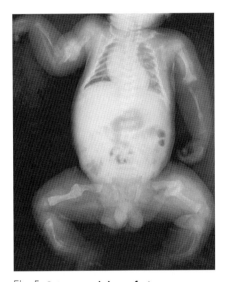

Fig. 5 **Osteogenesis imperfecta.** Demineralization with numerous fractures. Bone softening results in deformity.

associated with blue sclerae and islands of bone in the sutures of the skull (*Wormian bones*) (Fig. 4).

In the most severe forms, fractures occur in utero and after birth and may be multiple (Fig. 5). Occasionally, the multiple fractures occurring in children with this disease may be confused with those occurring in non-accidental injury. Usually the clinical context will differ.

Non-accidental injury

Violence to children may cause damage to the brain and abdominal viscera in the absence of evidence of skeletal trauma (in only 20–30% of cases of non-accidental injury (NAI) is evidence of skeletal trauma present).

Clinically, there may be external signs of NAI. If a bone lesion is

present, the child will be in pain and reluctant to use the part involved.

A skeletal survey is performed. Fractures may be seen at bone shafts, often at the ribs (Fig. 6). Multiple lesions are seen, of different generations. Some fractures will be healed, showing callus, others more recent. Skull fractures, often of different generations, may be present (Fig. 7), but brain damage, assessed at *computed tomography (CT) or magnetic resonance imaging (MRI)*, can occur in the absence of skull fracture (see p. 123).

Fractures of the shaft of a long bone may be transverse, across the long axis of a bone, after a direct blow, or spiral after a twisting or rotational injury.

The growth plate is a site of potential weakness and is a potential site of fracture in the immature skeleton (see p. 33).

In infants, a fracture through the growth plate will not show the displaced epiphysis if it is not yet

ossified, though soft-tissue deformity may well be present. Often, however, the displaced epiphysis takes with it a small flake of bone from the metaphyseal margin, a minor sign indicating major injury (the *Thurston Holland sign*) (Fig. 8). This is a Salter-Harris Type 2 lesion (see p. 33). The displaced cartilaginous epiphysis can be directly visualized with *ultrasound* or at *MRI*.

Elevation of the periosteum by haemorrhage gives a subsequent sheath of periosteal new bone (Fig. 8).

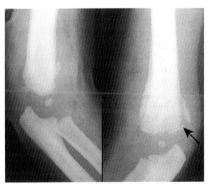

Fig. 8 **Non-accidental injury.** Displacement of a metaphyseal flake (arrow) and periosteal elevation due to haemorrhage.

Congenital disorders and non-accidental injury

Radiographic skeletal survey in the investigation of non-accidental injury

- Anteroposterior (AP) and lateral skull views – to include lateral cervical spine. Add Townes' view if there is occipital injury
- AP chest
- AP abdomen and pelvis
- Lateral thoracolumbar spine
- AP views of upper and lower limbs – include hands and feet
- Coned lateral views of knees and ankles if clinically suspicious.

Any neurologically unstable child requires cross-sectional brain imaging, or if a skull fracture has been seen on the plain film.

Generalized disorders

Haemolytic anaemia: sickle-cell disease and thalassaemia

Although often considered together, sickle-cell disease and thalassaemia have little in common radiologically. Thalassaemia gives the more severe bone disease as the anaemia is usually more severe.

Sickle-cell disease

Radiologically, changes relate to infarction in bone and avascular necrosis at joints. Red marrow cells die in the first day after the ischaemic episode, followed by osteoblasts, osteoclasts and fat cells. Marrow fibrosis and subsequent calcification result in patchy or diffuse osteosclerosis (Fig. 1). Sequestra may also be seen, especially linear sequestra relating to previous episodes of cortical necrosis (see p. 16).

At joints, changes similar to those in Perthes' disease of the hip result (see p. 27). Flattening, fragmentation and sclerosis of epiphyses occur with subsequent deformity. The joint space is preserved until secondary osteoarthritis supervenes.

Because of infarction, the bones are not expanded, with the exception of the skull vault (see below, under **thalassaemia**). The spleen, too, shrinks after infarction. With magnetic resonance imaging (MRI) the marrow in sickle-cell disease shows diminished signal due to changes of medullary

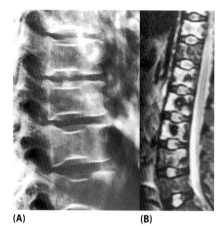

(A) **(B)**

Fig. 2 **Sickle-cell disease.** (A) The plain film of the spine shows well-demarcated, straight end-plate defects due to growth arrest following infarction of the central area of the vertebral body. The periphery of the body carries on growing, however, as its blood supply derives from local perforating vessels. (B) Magnetic resonance imaging of the spine shows the centrally infarcted area, seen as low signal change.

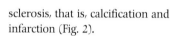

sclerosis, that is, calcification and infarction (Fig. 2).

Thalassaemia

Marrow hypertrophy occurs in an attempt to replenish red blood cells, which have a shortened life. Radiologically, this results in bone expansion, cortical thinning and diminution of medullary trabeculation (Fig. 3). Bones thus appear osteopenic, but with residual, rather coarsened trabeculation.

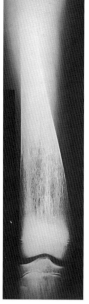

Fig. 4 **Thalassaemia.** An 'Erlenmeyer flask' appearance of femur is seen.

Bone expansion at metaphyses gives a so-called *Erlenmeyer flask* appearance (Fig. 4).

Thickening of the skull vault appears in association with a spiculated *hair-on-end* appearance, as new bone is laid down on stretched Sharpey's fibres, which connect the pericranium to the skull vault (Fig. 5). This occurs to a lesser extent in sickle-cell disease.

The paranasal air sinuses are also obliterated by marrow, with the exception of the ethmoid.

Extramedullary haemopoiesis occurs, giving an *enlarged* liver or spleen. Iron deposition occurs in the

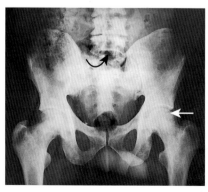

Fig. 1 **Sickle-cell disease.** Uniform sclerosis of the spine, pelvis and proximal femora in a patient with multifocal bone infarcts. There is also early collapse of the left femoral head (arrow). Degenerative changes are seen in the lumbar spine together with end-plate defects (curved arrows).

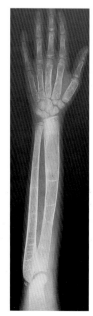

Fig. 3 **Thalassaemia.** Expansion of the marrow results in broadening of the bones, especially at their ends. Cortical thinning results.

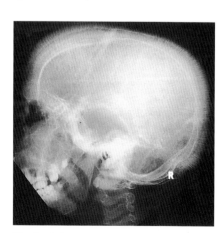

Fig. 5 **Thalassaemia – marrow hyperplasia and extramedullary haemopoiesis.** The paranasal air sinuses become obliterated and the skull vault thickens. Elevation of the pericranium results in new bone being laid down upon the stretched Sharpey's fibres, seen as a 'hair on end' appearance.

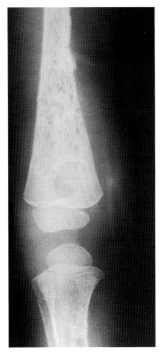

Fig. 6 **Gaucher's disease.** An Erlenmeyer flask appearance with multifocal lytic change, the result of Gaucher cell deposition in bone.

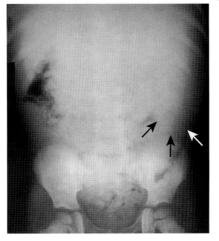

Fig. 7 **Gaucher's disease.** Deposition of Gaucher cells results in splenomegaly (arrows).

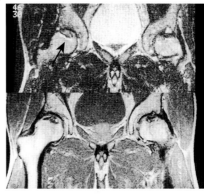

Fig. 8 **Avascular necrosis** – T1 (top) and T2-weighted (bottom) magnetic resonance images (MRI). Symmetrical femoral head collapse is demonstrated, together with cyst formation in the femoral heads and low signal change in and around the areas of necrosis (arrow), which would be seen as increased density or calcification on a plain film. The changes seen at MRI mirror those seen on the plain film.

soft tissues due to excess red blood cell breakdown. This can be assessed at *MR examination* due to the signal void or depletion caused by iron.

Gaucher's disease

This is another inherited disorder due to an enzyme defect and is commoner in Jews. Large amounts of a lipid, *glucosylceramide*, are laid down in bone and soft tissues.

Radiologically, splenomegaly and an *Erlenmeyer flask* appearance are seen. The bony deposits cause focal osteolytic lesions (Fig. 6). Compression of intraosseous blood vessels by the abnormal Gaucher cells results in bone infarction and articular avascular necrosis.

Marrow infiltration also causes low signal change at MRI, as well as those of avascular necrosis and bone infarction.

Radiologically, these diseases are all adequately imaged using *conventional plain films* for assessing bone change. Visceromegaly due to extramedullary haemopoiesis may be seen on *plain films* (Fig. 7) or with *ultrasound, CT or MRI*, which also show soft-tissue extramedullary haemopoiesis.

Avascular necrosis

Plain film changes have been previously described in the sections on

Perthes' disease and sickle-cell disease (see p. 27).

CT to assess bone changes at joints in chronic avascular necrosis is often used prior to joint replacement.

MRI is the examination of choice to assess marrow change in bone in avascular necrosis. Oedema in the avascular area and hyperaemia in the surrounding bone cause characteristic change. When oedema replaces fat in marrow, the signal increases in T2-weighted sequences and decreases on T1-weighting (Fig. 8). Hyperaemia in surrounding bone results in peripheral signal increase (and increased uptake on a *radionuclide bone scan*, which also shows photopenia in the avascular area).

Subsequent fibrosis and necrosis in the marrow with calcification cause signal loss. The margin of the avascular area becomes well-defined by a low signal serpiginous band, sometimes associated with an adjacent very bright parallel double line (Fig. 8).

Plain films also show marginal sclerosis around the avascular area. This 'zone of creeping substitution' lies at the margin of the advancing front of revascularization around the infarct.

Box 1 Causes of avascular necrosis

Traumatic
- Fracture
- Radiation therapy
- Thermal injury.

Inflammatory
- Collagen disorders, e.g. systemic lupus erythematosus
- Rheumatoid arthritis
- Septic arthritis.

Metabolic
- Cushing's syndrome.

Haematological
- Haemoglobinopathies
- Haemophilia
- Gaucher's disease.

Iatrogenic
- Steroid therapy
- Antimitotic drugs.

Idiopathic
- Perthes' disease.

Generalized disorders

Radiological investigation of avascular necrosis
- Plain films – show bone changes
- Computed tomography – assesses changes at joints
- Radioisotope bone scanning shows photopenia in the affected bone initially, but increased uptake with healing
- Magnetic resonance imaging shows changes in marrow, both in acute and chronic phases, as well as the end-stage bony deformity.

Trauma: general considerations

A fracture is defined as a breach or interruption in the continuity of a bone which occurs when an abnormal force acts on a normal or abnormal bone, or when a normal force acts on abnormal bone.

A force is the push or pull acting on a body that tends to deform that body (Fig. 1). *Stress* is the initial reaction or force generated within a body to an external force applied to it. *Strain* is change occurring in the linear dimensions of a body on the application of a force and may be *tensile, compressive* or *shearing*.

Children's bones are less mineralized than adults and can absorb more energy before they fracture. Their bones are more plastic.

The pattern of a fracture depends on the nature and direction of the deforming force.

Fractures may be caused by direct or indirect trauma.

Indirect trauma

This is defined as having been caused by forces acting at a distance from the fracture site:

Transverse or angulation fractures
With progressive angulation, fibres under tension fail progressively towards the centre of a bone, while

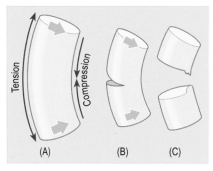

Fig. 2 **Transverse fractures** of bone result from progressive angulation. Bone under compression splinters on the concave side.

those under compression splinter. The resulting transverse fracture has minor comminution on the concavity (Fig. 2).

Spiral or rotational fractures
A rotational stress applied at the end of a long bone causes a spiral fracture at 45° to the long axis of the bone with a shear deformity.

Oblique fractures
These are caused by angulation and vertical loading. The greater the angulation on the concavity, the greater the obliquity (Figs 3 & 4).

True traction or avulsion fractures
These are transverse fractures produced at sites of tendinous insertion. Apophyses are commonly avulsed in children.

Vertical compression – axial loading
Usually the shaft of a long bone is driven down into the wider bone end,

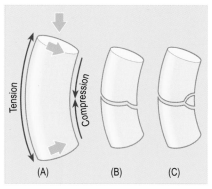

Fig. 4 (A) **Angulation plus vertical compression** results in a transverse fracture on the side under tension, continuing into an oblique fracture line on the side under compression (B). (C) The oblique segment then shears off to give a butterfly segment.

giving a 'Y'-shaped fracture (Fig. 5). Vertical compression lesions also cause comminution of vertebral bodies.

Greenstick fracture
This occurs usually in children whose bones are plastic. The energy is sufficient to begin the fracture but not to apply it across the entire bone. Shear cracks open up within the bone preventing transverse propagation of the fracture (Fig. 6A).

Torus or buckle fracture
This is a slight buckling of the cortex of one side of a bone (Fig. 6B). Often greenstick and torus fractures occur together.

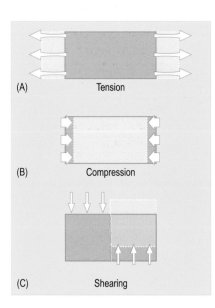

Fig. 1 **Three types of force** acting on a body are demonstrated. Tension elongates a body, compression shortens a body and shearing causes movement of one part over another.

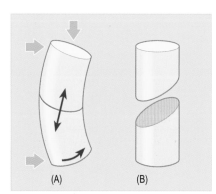

Fig. 3 **Oblique fracture.** (A) Angulation plus vertical loading is applied to a bone in association with rotation. (B) An oblique fracture results with blunt, rounded, smooth margins.

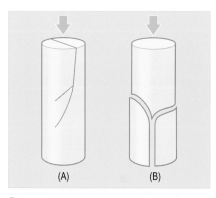

Fig. 5 **Vertical compression.** (A) A vertical or vertical-oblique fracture theoretically results. (B) More often, however, the shaft is driven down into the wider metaphysis, which then fragments, giving a 'Y' fracture.

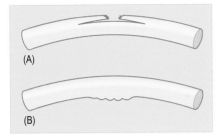

Fig. 6 (A) **Greenstick fracture.** The bone is bowed and the cortex is incompletely fractured around part of the circumference. (B) **Torus fracture.** Bowing of the bone is associated with a buckled, rather than fractured, cortex on the concavity.

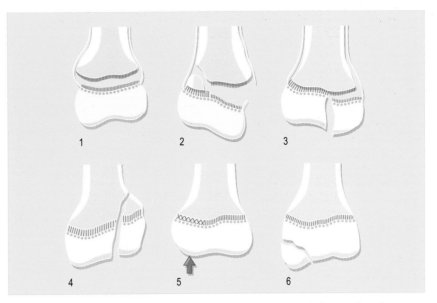

Fig. 7 **Salter-Harris classification of fractures around the epiphyseal plate.** (Adapted from Salter & Harris 1963 Injuries involving the epiphyseal plate. Journal of Bone and Joint Surgery 45A: 587–622)

Direct trauma

These injuries are more easily understood. The changes are due to direct application of a force to bone, such as penetrating injury or a direct crush injury.

In children fractures are described in relation to the epiphysis, the growth plate or *physis*, and the metaphysis or the diaphysis. The presence, in childhood, of the cartilaginous growth plate leads to an increased incidence of local fractures in childhood. Some 15–20% of fractures in children occur at the growth plate and epiphysis. Fractures through the growth plate have been classified according to the alignment of the fracture line (Fig. 7). These fractures may result in premature growth plate fusion, shortening and deformity.

In adult life, fractures may be described as articular, subarticular or in the upper, middle or lower thirds of the shaft of a long bone.

Stress fracture

Repeated submaximal forces act at specific sites during specific activity. The bone eventually gives way, but pain occurs before the fracture becomes visible. A 'march' fracture in the metatarsal of a soldier is the classic example.

Pain is initially associated with abnormal radioisotope bone scans and magnetic resonance (MR) images – the latter will show the fracture line before it is visible on the plain film.

Subsequent films show the fracture, the deformity and callus. Pain relief is obtained by cessation of the causative physical activity.

Soft-tissue changes and fracture

Fractures and dislocations are inevitably associated with local soft tissue abnormality. As a generalization, it can be said that in the absence of clinically evident soft-tissue swelling, a fracture is extremely unlikely to be present. Soft tissues may indicate the presence of an underlying bone or soft-tissue injury, and can be seen both clinically and radiologically.

Fractures are associated with bleeding into surrounding soft tissues, which displaces local fat planes. These are particularly evident over joints – the elbow, knee, wrist and ankle. In addition, intra-articular fractures release medullary fat into the joint space, where it floats on released blood. A horizontal X-ray beam then demonstrates an intra-articular fat-fluid level.

Soft-tissue haemorrhage and effusions are also demonstrated with *ultrasound*.

MRI is especially useful in demonstrating soft-tissue change, as well as fractures and interosseous bone oedema or bruising, and effusions.

Fractures are also well demonstrated using radionuclide bone scanning, much increase in uptake of isotope being seen. This investigation is very sensitive.

Fractures may be difficult to determine in the elderly osteoporotic patient if there is little or no displacement of fracture parts. The absence of trabeculation makes visualization of the fracture difficult. While radionuclide bone scanning and computed tomography (CT) are useful tools in the diagnosis of these latent fractures, MRI is both sensitive and specific in their diagnosis.

Individual fractures are dealt with in the companion textbook of this series (McRae R, Kinninmonth AWG 1997 Orthopaedics and trauma. Churchill Livingstone, Edinburgh).

Trauma

Radiological investigation of fractures
- A significance percentage of fractures in children occur around the growth plate
- Fractures in children may be difficult to visualize
- Children's bones are soft and bow
- Fractures are difficult to visualize in the elderly osteoporotic skeleton
- Fractures are always associated with local soft-tissue swelling.

Respiratory System

Acute chest pain 1

Chest pain and breathlessness are two of the most common symptoms that present to a medical practitioner at all stages of his or her career. It is with this in mind that we would like to present a practical approach to understanding the radiology of the important conditions that may present this way.

Acute chest pain

The main objective when confronted with a patient with acute chest pain is to confirm or exclude potentially lethal causes of pain. The most important of these causes are summarized in Box 1.

Unstable angina

Unstable angina is defined as angina occurring at rest or on minimal exertion, without the electrocardiogram (ECG) or enzyme changes of a myocardial infarction (MI). Angina represents myocardial ischaemia and is almost always secondary to coronary artery disease.

Rarer causes include aortic stenosis, severe arrhythmias (causing hypoperfusion) and anaemia. Characteristically, the patient presents with central crushing chest pain, which may radiate to the jaw and one or both arms. The ECG is often normal between

> **Box 1 Causes of acute chest pain**
>
> - Unstable angina
> - Myocardial infarction
> - Pneumothorax
> - Pulmonary emboli
> - Aortic dissection
> - Oesophageal rupture

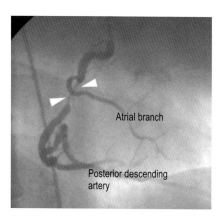

Fig. 1 **Coronary angiography.** There is a tight stricture of the right coronary artery (arrowheads).

attacks, although ST segment depression and flattening, or T wave inversion, may signify ischaemia.

The chest X-ray (CXR) is often normal, but is a useful adjunct in

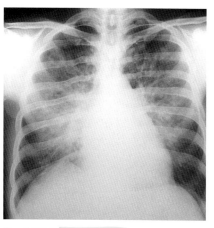

Fig. 2 **Pulmonary oedema** – bilateral peri-hilar airspace shadowing. Fluid fills the alveoli, the result of pulmonary venous hypertension.

excluding other causes of pain. A coronary arteriogram usually demonstrates atherosclerotic narrowing in the coronary artery circulation (Fig. 1).

Myocardial infarction

MI is defined as the irreversible necrosis of cardiac muscle secondary to coronary artery disease. Chest pain is usually of greater severity and duration than in angina, and may be associated with extreme anxiety, sweating and vomiting. The patient is often distressed, cold, clammy, tachycardic, hypertensive or hypotensive. Characteristic ECG changes are ST segment elevation in the leads adjacent to the infarct along with elevation of cardiac enzymes.

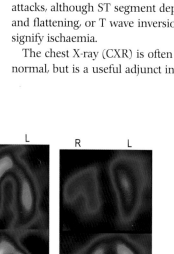

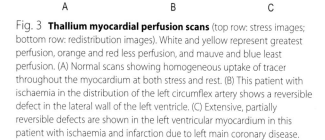

Fig. 3 **Thallium myocardial perfusion scans** (top row: stress images; bottom row: redistribution images). White and yellow represent greatest perfusion, orange and red less perfusion, and mauve and blue least perfusion. (A) Normal scans showing homogeneous uptake of tracer throughout the myocardium at both stress and rest. (B) This patient with ischaemia in the distribution of the left circumflex artery shows a reversible defect in the lateral wall of the left ventricle. (C) Extensive, partially reversible defects are shown in the left ventricular myocardium in this patient with ischaemia and infarction due to left main coronary disease.

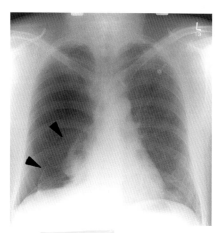

Fig. 4 **Pneumothorax.** The edge of the right lung is clearly visible with no lung markings seen peripheral to the edge (arrowheads).

The chest X-ray may be normal, but may demonstrate complications such as pulmonary oedema (Fig. 2) or an alternative pathology such as an aortic dissection.

Radionuclide thallium scanning is a form of functional imaging that is used to differentiate ischaemic from infarcted myocardium (Fig. 3).

Pneumothorax

Pneumothorax is defined as an accumulation of air in the pleural space. This is often spontaneous (usually in tall thin men) due to rupture of a pleural bleb. It may be traumatic, iatrogenic (following invasive procedures or mechanical ventilation), or a complication of asthma or chronic obstructive pulmonary disease (COPD). The clinical features include sudden dyspnoea and pleuritic chest pain. It may be classified as a 'simple' pneumothorax, when there is no associated mediastinal shift, or a 'tension' pneumothorax, if there is associated mediastinal shift away from the side of the pneumothorax.

On the CXR look for a 'lung edge' with an area devoid of lung markings peripheral to the edge of the lung (Fig. 4). This may be very subtle and may be better visualized on an expiratory film, where the constant volume of air in the pneumothorax is increased relative to the amount in the lung in expiration. CT of the chest is infrequently used as an adjunct in difficult cases, and demonstrates features exactly similar to those on the CXR (Fig. 5).

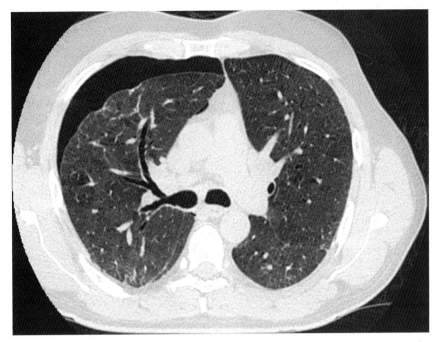

Fig. 5 **Pneumothorax.** The CT demonstrates the same features as on the chest X-ray; the edge of the right pneumothorax is clearly visible.

Acute chest pain 1

Suspected cause	Imaging technique
Unstable angina	Chest X-ray (CXR)
	Coronary arteriogram
Myocardial infarction	CXR
	Radionuclide thalium scan
Pneumothorax	CXR
	Computed tomography (CT) thorax
Pulmonary embolus	CXR
	Lung ventilation – perfusion (VQ) scan
	CT pulmonary angiography (CTPA)
	Conventional pulmonary angiography (PA)
Aortic dissection	CXR
	Contrast enhanced CT
	Magnetic resonance angiography (MRA)
	Ultrasound (US)
Oesophageal rupture	CXR
	Water soluble swallow
	CT thorax.

Acute chest pain 2: pulmonary embolus, aortic dissection and oesophageal rupture

Pulmonary embolus

Pulmonary embolus (PE) is defined as the passage of thrombus, usually from the systemic venous circulation, into the pulmonary arterial circulation occluding blood flow to the lungs. Characteristic presentation is one of acute breathlessness associated with pleuritic chest pain and occasional haemoptysis. The patient is usually hypoxic, but the classical electrocardiogram (ECG) changes are only seen in a massive embolus. A pulmonary embolus should always be suspected if a patient collapses suddenly 1–2 weeks after surgery, since this may be due to movement of a clot following a deep vein thrombosis in the calf or thigh.

The chest X-ray is often normal. There may be decreased vascular markings due to vascular occlusion, an elevated hemidiaphragm, a small pleural effusion or focal shadowing. The classic *Hampton's hump* (Fig. 1) – a peripheral wedge-shaped area of infarction, is only seen in 1–2%. The chest X-ray is principally of value in excluding alternative diagnoses (e.g. myocardial infarction, pneumonia and pneumothorax).

In a VQ scan the main abnormality suggestive of a pulmonary embolus is one of 'VQ mismatch', i.e. an abnormality of perfusion against a background of normal ventilation (Fig. 2). If, however, the patient has pre-existing lung disease or the presenting chest X-ray is abnormal, there is a high likelihood of abnormal ventilation resulting in defects in both ventilation **and** perfusion. Hence, the overall sensitivity of the investigation is reduced. However this limitation has been overcome with the advent of CT pulmonary angiography (CTPA).

CTPA is of particular use in those with pre-existing lung disease, and aims to actually detect filling defects (representing emboli) within the pulmonary vascular bed (Fig. 3).

PA is the 'gold standard' investigation, but is usually only performed in specialized centres. Its use has declined significantly, particularly with the advent of CTPA.

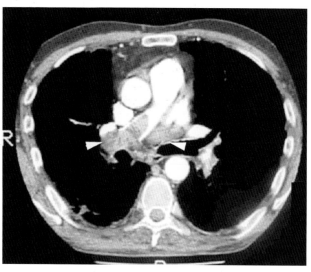

Fig. 3 **Pulmonary emboli** – computed tomography pulmonary angiogram (CTPA). Large filling defects (arrowheads), representing emboli (grey), are seen in the main pulmonary arteries, which are opacified by contrast medium (white).

Aortic dissection

Dissecting aneurysms are mainly encountered in the aorta. Hypertension is the main predisposing factor and men are mostly affected, usually aged between 50 and 70 years. Only 5% of cases are under 40 years and are usually associated with an underlying abnormality, such as Marfan's syndrome.

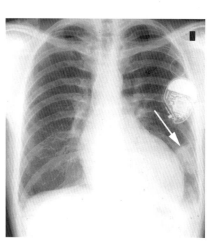

Fig. 1 **Pulmonary infarction.** A peripheral wedge-shaped 'Hampton's hump' is seen in the left lower lobe (arrow).

Fig. 2 **Pulmonary embolism.** The scan demonstrates 'V/Q' mismatch, an abnormality of perfusion (Q) against a background of normal ventilation (V).

V

Q

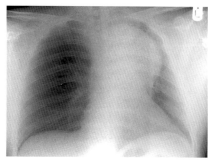

Fig. 4 **Aortic dissection.** Widening of the superior mediastinum is seen due to haemorrhage.

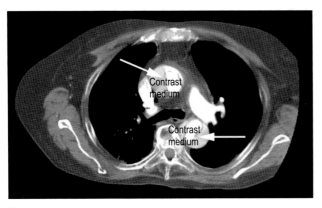

Fig. 5 **Type A aortic dissection.** The dissection flap (arrows) is visible in both the ascending and descending aortas.

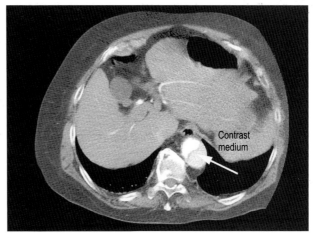

Fig. 6 **Type B aortic dissection.** The 'tennis ball' sign is seen in the descending aorta.

The underlying aetiology is usually due to cystic medial degeneration of the vessel wall. Dissections usually commence in the aortic arch or ascending aorta and extend distally. The clinical features include sudden onset of severe inter-scapular chest or upper abdominal pain, asymmetry of the peripheral pulses, unequal blood pressure in both arms and associated neurological symptoms – such as transient ischaemic attack (TIA) or stroke.

Mediastinal widening is shown on the chest X-ray, but this can be very difficult to assess in these sick patients due to the magnification factor that occurs with anteroposterior (AP) chest films (as they are often obtained with the patient sitting or supine) (Fig. 4).

Contrast-enhanced computed tomography (CT) is now the investigation of choice in suspected aortic dissection. Look for a dissection flap within the aortic lumen – forming the so-called 'tennis ball' sign.

Aortic dissection is usually classified as either type A (involves the Ascending aorta) or type B (**B**elow the arch of aorta) (Figs 5 & 6).

Oesophageal rupture

Oesophageal rupture may occur spontaneously following a bout of vomiting, be caused by oesophageal instrumentation or be caused by the swallowing of a sharp foreign body. Clinical features are of severe chest or epigastric pain.

On the plain chest X-ray there may be mediastinal air, a pleural effusion

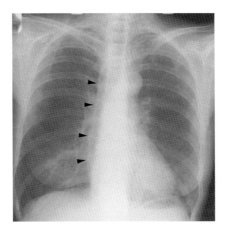

Fig. 7 **Oesophageal rupture.** Air is seen outlining the right side of the mediastinum (arrowheads).

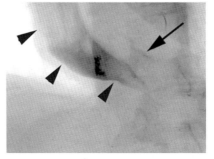

Fig. 8 **Water-soluble swallow.** This demonstrates the leak of contrast medium (arrow) from the distal third of the oesophagus (arrowheads).

or mediastinal widening (secondary to a haematoma) (Fig. 7).

A water-soluble contrast swallow demonstrates extravasation of contrast from the oesophagus (Fig. 8).

CT of the thorax will demonstrate a left-sided pleural effusion and occasionally the defect in the oesophageal wall (see Box 1 for additional chest pain causes).

> ### Box 1 Other causes of acute chest pain
>
> **Common**
> - Gastro-oesophageal reflux
> - Rib fractures, costochondritis
> - Pericarditis
> - Pleurisy.
>
> **Uncommon**
> - Varicella zoster
> - Ankylosing spondylitis
> - Tabes dorsalis
> - Gallbladder and pancreatic disease.

> ### Pulmonary embolus, aortic dissection and oesophageal rupture
>
> - A routine chest X-ray in pulmonary embolus is often normal, but excludes other diagnoses.
> - A chest X-ray in aortic dissection is usually abnormal – the mediastinum is widened and there may be a collection of fluid, usually at the left lung base.
> - Oesophageal rupture may also have an abnormal chest X-ray, again with evidence of mediastinal widening and a pleural effusion.

Acute breathlessness 1

The main objective is to rapidly assess for the more common causes of breathlessness and initiate early treatment. The most important of these causes are outlined in Box 1 and additional causes are listed in Box 2.

Asthma

Bronchospasm occurs most commonly in an atopic individual, who may have eczema, hayfever, allergies, or in those with a family history of asthma. Clinical features are of acute breathlessness with an associated wheeze.

The chest X-ray may be normal. However, in chronic cases of asthma the lungs may be hyperinflated (Fig. 1).

> **Box 1 Causes of acute breathlessness**
>
> - Asthma
> - Pulmonary oedema
> - Pneumonia
> - Acute exacerbation chronic obstructive pulmonary disease
> - Pulmonary embolism
> - Pneumothorax.

> **Box 2 Other causes of acute breathlessness**
>
> - Cardiac tamponade
> - Tracheobronchial obstruction
> - Laryngeal obstruction.

Occasionally, complications may be visible on the chest film, e.g. pneumothorax or infection.

Pulmonary oedema

This may be cardiogenic or non-cardiogenic. Cardiogenic pulmonary oedema results from high pulmonary venous pressure – a consequence of myocardial disease, cardiac valvular disease or fluid overload (e.g. post transfusion or renal failure). Non-cardiogenic pulmonary oedema results

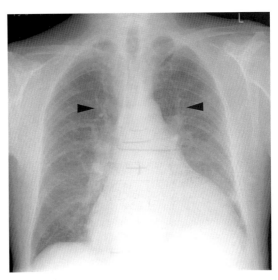

Fig. 2 **Raised pulmonary venous pressure.** There is cardiomegaly with redistribution of pulmonary blood flow to both upper lobes (arrowheads). This is termed 'upper lobe blood diversion'.

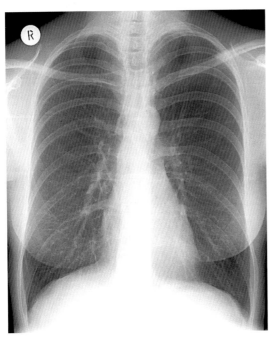

Fig. 1 **Asthma.** The lungs are hyperinflated but the lung parenchyma and mediastinal contour appear normal.

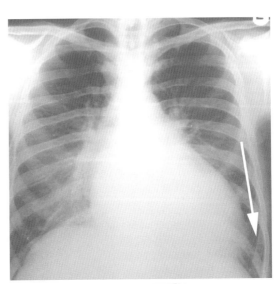

Fig. 3 **Interstitial pulmonary oedema.** Upper lobe blood diversion and the formation of 'septal lines' (short, horizontally orientated lines extending to pleura, perpendicular to pleura in costophrenic angles) at the left costophrenic angle.

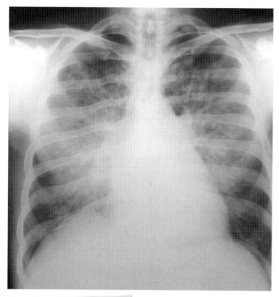

Fig. 4 **Pulmonary oedema.** Bilateral peri-hilar airspace shadowing is demonstrated.

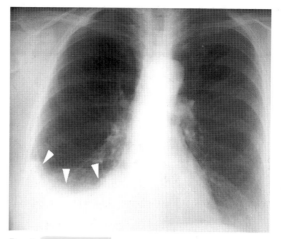

Fig. 5 **Pleural effusion.** A meniscus-shaped collection of fluid is shown at the right base (arrowheads).

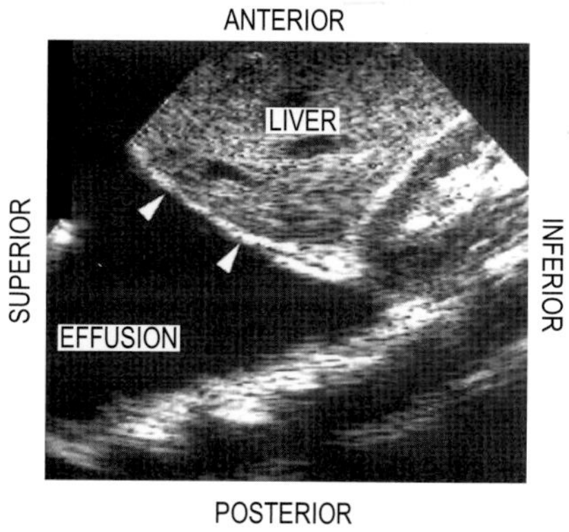

Fig. 6 **Simple pleural effusion** – ultrasound. The arrowheads denote the position of the diaphragm.

from an increase in pulmonary capillary permeability as in adult respiratory distress syndrome (ARDS).

Clinical features are acute dyspnoea, a cough, with or without pink frothy sputum, orthopnoea and paroxysmal nocturnal dyspnoea.

There is a spectrum of radiological features on the plain chest film, ranging from redistribution of blood flow from lower to upper zones in the erect position, which indicates pulmonary venous hypertension (Fig. 2), progressing on to interstitial oedema (Fig. 3) prior to developing alveolar pulmonary oedema (Fig. 4). Pleural effusions may also be caused by heart failure (Figs 5 & 6).

Echocardiography may be performed if valvular disease is suspected as a contributory cause for heart failure.

Pleural effusion

On an anterior view radiograph, a pleural effusion is seen as a meniscus rising up in the axillary line. In fact, it is of equal height all the way round the pleural space, but because of the increased density of the fluid in the axillary line, it appears more prominent there. A lateral view would show exactly the opposite, that is, fluid anteriorly and posteriorly, but not in the mid portion of the lung base.

The appearance may be understood by thinking of two sheets of glass standing in a water bath. The water creeps up between the two sheets of glass, which represent the visceral and parietal pleura.

Effusions may result from local pathology within the pleura, such as tumour or infection, which increase permeability of the pleura. They may also be due to an increased pulmonary venous pressure, which increases microvascular pressure in the lungs, causing fluid to accumulate in the pleura.

Acute breathlessness 1

Radiological investigation
- Asthma: chest X-ray (CXR)
- Pulmonary oedema: CXR, echocardiography
- Pneumonia: CXR
- Chronic obstructive pulmonary disease: CXR.

Acute breathlessness 2: pneumonia and chronic obstructive pulmonary disease

Pneumonia

Pneumonia may be classified on the basis of the aetiology (Box 1) (an aetiological factor being found in 75% of patients) or anatomically – e.g. lobar (Box 2) and non-lobar pneumonias (Box 3).

Complications of pneumonia

The most significant complications are those of lung abscess formation (Fig. 1), and the development of an empyema (Fig. 2). A lung abscess may develop following *Staphylococcus aureus* and *Klebsiella pneumoniae* infection. An empyema refers to the presence of pus within the pleural space, following either the rupture of a lung abscess into the pleural cavity or from bacterial spread from a severe pneumonia.

Chronic obstructive pulmonary disease

Chronic obstructive pulmonary disease (COPD) is a label that covers a number of different diagnoses, including emphysema, chronic bronchitis, chronic obstructive airways disease and chronic asthma. COPD, therefore, is not a disease itself, rather a syndrome encompassing a number of different diseases.

COPD is usually linked with chronic cigarette smoking of over 20 years of duration and patients usually present in middle age with a chest infection or repeated episodes of coughing and productive sputum. Patients are usually short of breath on exertion (SOBOE) and may often wheeze on forced expiration.

In emphysema the lungs are over-inflated and are of large volume. The diaphragms are low and flat. There is little movement between inspiration and expiration. The alveoli distal to the terminal bronchioles are destroyed permanently. Emphysema is defined pathologically as 'dilatation and destruction of lung parenchyma distal to the terminal bronchioles'. Cigarette smoking is a major factor in the development of both chronic bronchitis and emphysema.

Chronic bronchitis is defined as 'sputum production on most days for 3 months of the year, for 2 or more consecutive years'. The bronchial walls are thickened, especially at the lung bases, and there is an increased amount of bronchial secretion. Upper-zone blood diversion may be seen as a result of emphysematous changes in the lung bases.

Box 1 Aetiological classification of pneumonia

Community acquired
- *Streptococcus pneumoniae*
- *Mycoplasma pneumoniae*
- *Staphylococcus aureus*
- Influenza A virus

Hospital acquired
- Gram-negative organisms

Box 2 Causes of lobar pneumonia

- *Streptococcus pneumoniae* – usually unilobar consolidation
- *Klebsiella pneumoniae* – usually causes multilobar consolidation with associated lobar enlargement and cavitation
- *Staphylococcus aureus* – especially in children
- Tuberculosis (TB) – in primary or post primary TB.

Box 3 Causes of non-lobar pneumonia

- *Haemophilus influenzae* – particularly in pre-existing lung disease, e.g. chronic obstructive pulmonary disease.
- *Pseudomonas aeruginosa* – especially in patients with cystic fibrosis.
- *Pneumocystis carinii* – in the immunocompromised patient
- Atypical pneumonias – *Mycoplasma*, *Chlamydia* and *Coxiella burnetti*.

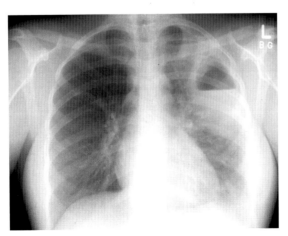

Fig. 1 **Cavitating pneumonia.** A thick-walled abscess is seen with an air-fluid level in the left upper lobe.

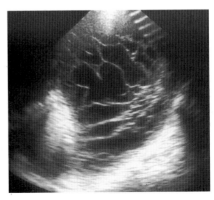

Fig. 2 **Empyema** – ultrasound. A heavily septated effusion is demonstrated. Note its complex nature and the difference compared to the simple effusion shown in Fig. 6 p. 41.

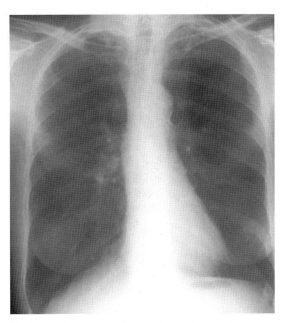

Fig. 3 **Emphysema.** The lungs are hyperinflated with flattening of both hemidiaphragms.

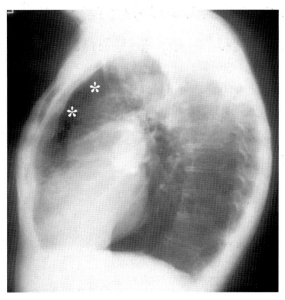

Fig. 4 **Emphysema** – lateral chest radiograph. There is a barrel-shaped chest with an increased retrosternal air space (asterisks). Note the flattened diaphragm.

The radiological features of COPD include the presence of lung bullae, severe hyperinflation of the lungs (more than 6 anterior ribs clearly visible above the diaphragm), in association with flattened diaphragms (Fig. 3) and a large retrosternal airspace seen on a lateral view (Fig. 4). There may be evidence of pneumonia on these background changes.

Two other causes of breathlessness have already been discussed – **pulmonary embolism** on page 38 and **pneumothorax** on page 37.

Sites of consolidation

Consolidation of the lung occurs when the terminal airspaces fill with fluid or solid material. This may be due to infective exudate or oedema fluid. Patent airways surrounded by the non-aerated lung appear as dark branching structures within the white, solid lung. This is called an 'air bronchogram'.

On the normal chest X-ray (CXR) the heart is outlined by aerated lung. If the lung adjacent to the heart becomes consolidated, it will have the same radiographic density as the heart, and that part of the heart border will appear indistinct or invisible. So, for example, consolidation of the right middle lobe (which lies against the right heart border) will obscure the right heart border (see Fig. 5), and consolidation in the lingula will obscure the left heart border. This is known as the 'silhouette sign'.

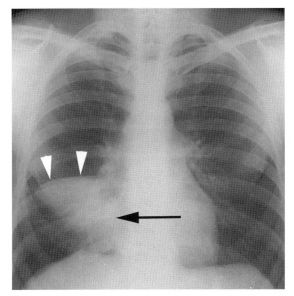
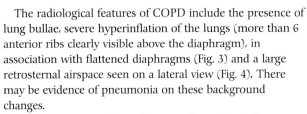

Fig. 5 **Infection.** Consolidation of the right middle lobe abuts the horizontal fissure (arrowheads) with effacement of the right heart border (arrow).

> ### Pneumonia and chronic obstructive pulmonary disease
>
> - Different types of pneumonia have different radiological appearances.
> - *Streptococcus pneumoniae* is usually unilobar, while tuberculosis may well be apical.
> - Immune-suppressed patients get opportunistic infections.
> - In emphysema the lungs are over-inflated with low flat diaphragms and a thin narrow vertical heart.
> - Chronic obstructive pulmonary disease is related to cigarette smoking and the lung markings are generally increased due to the changes of chronic bronchitis, bronchial wall thickening and increased perfusion.

Chronic cough, chest pain, haemoptysis and breathlessness 1

The important differential diagnoses to consider in this group are listed in Box 1.

Bronchogenic carcinoma, secondary lung tumours and granulomatous lung disease are discussed in the following pages.

Differentiation between malignant and benign lung tumours

Benign tumours do not grow rapidly or significantly under radiological observation. This is not the case for malignant lesions unless they have been or are being treated. Malignant tumours are also usually larger than benign lesions and, because they infiltrate the surrounding tissues, they are more likely to be irregular than benign tumours, which tend to have a smooth margin.

Calcification is not a feature of malignant tumours in the lung but is seen with benign lesions.

When a malignant tumour erodes into a bronchus, its contents are coughed up and reciprocally air enters the now cavitating tumour mass. An air-fluid level may be seen. Malignant cavities are usually thick walled, though squamous cell carcinomas may have a thin wall.

Lymphoma
Lymphoma is a proliferative disorder of the lymphoreticular system. Malignant lymphomas may be subdivided into two groups: *Hodgkin's disease* and a group of *non-Hodgkin's*

lymphomas. Hodgkin's disease is more common in the thorax than non-Hodgkin's disease.

The clinical features include enlarged cervical lymph nodes, a fever with drenching night sweats and weight loss.

Mediastinal and hilar adenopathy is the most common manifestation, present in 90–99%. Hilar nodes are involved bilaterally in 50% (Fig. 1).

Pancoast tumour
Pancoast tumour is a bronchial carcinoma arising at the lung apex. The ribs, spine and spinal cord, as well as brachial plexus and local sympathetic nerves may be invaded. The X-ray, therefore, shows a tumour mass with adjacent bone destruction. These changes are better visualised at

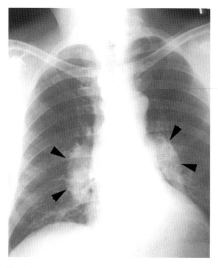

Fig. 1 **Hodgkin's disease.** There is bilateral hilar adenopathy (arrowheads).

cross-sectional imaging by computed tomography (CT) or magnetic resonance imaging (MRI).

Distant symptoms of primary malignant tumours

Hypertrophic osteoarthropathy
Patients present with bone and joint pain. Radiological examination shows lamellar periostitis of the long bones of the hands and forearms especially, but also of the tibia, fibula and foot (Fig. 2). A radioisotope bone scan is strongly positive with a linear distribution of increased uptake along the cortex of the affected bone.

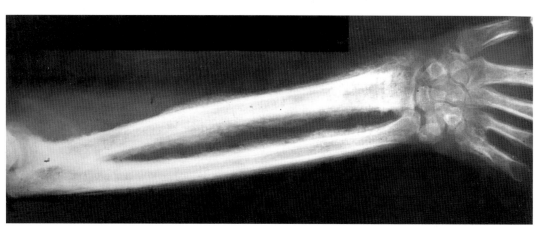

Fig. 2 **Hypertrophic osteoarthropathy.**
A shaggy periostitis is seen along the radius and ulna. The carpal bones are not affected but the metacarpals are.

These changes are not only seen with lung disease but can also occur with chronic gastrointestinal disease.

Removal of the malignant tumour often results in resolution of the painful periostitis.

Fibrosing lung disease

Whatever the aetiology, diffuse fibrosing lung disease (Box 2) may cause progressive dyspnoea, dry cough and fatigue (over 1–5 years), with restrictive pulmonary function tests. The distribution of radiographic changes is a characteristically *basal predominance*.

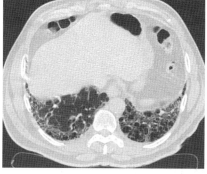

Fig. 4   **Chronic fibrosing alveolitis** – high-resolution computed tomography scan. Coarse reticular bibasal fibrosis resembling 'honeycombing' is demonstrated.

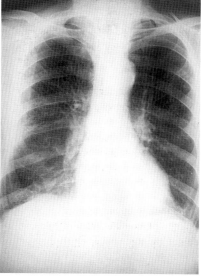

(A)

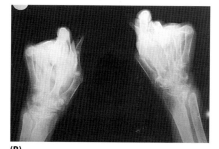

(B)

Fig. 5   **Interstitial fibrosis in rheumatoid arthritis.** (A) Extensive interstitial linear added shadowing is demonstrated in both lungfields with relative sparing of the apices. There is pulmonary arterial hypertension, as shown by prominence of the hilar shadows. (B) The hands in this patient demonstrate gross deformity due to chronic rheumatoid arthritis. Note the erosions of the distal ulna and radius.

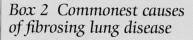

Box 2 Commonest causes of fibrosing lung disease

- Cryptogenic fibrosing alveolitis (CFA)
- Connective-tissue disease
  - Rheumatoid lung
  - Systemic sclerosis.

Cryptogenic fibrosing alveolitis

This is the commonest (90%) form of idiopathic interstitial pneumonitis.

The chext X-ray may demonstrate bilateral diffuse linear or small irregular reticular opacities predominantly at the lung bases (85%). Honeycombing may be seen in advanced disease (in up to 74%) with progressive loss of lung volume (Fig. 3).

High resolution CT (HRCT) characteristically shows reticular

shadowing with a predominantly basal and subpleural distribution. The reticular shadowing may be coarse and resemble honeycombs (Fig. 4).

Connective-tissue disease

Rheumatoid lung

Fibrosing lung disease occurs in up to 50% of patients with rheumatoid arthritis with a male predominance (M:F=5:1) (Fig. 5). This is in contradistinction to rheumatoid arthritis in general, which has a female predominance (RA F>>M).

Systemic sclerosis

This is a multisystem connective-tissue disorder of unknown aetiology. Pulmonary involvement occurs in 10–25%.

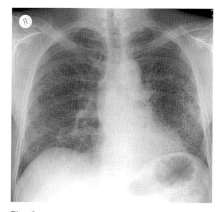

Fig. 3   **Chronic fibrosing alveolitis.** Diffuse bilateral linear and small irregular reticulations with a basal predominance are demonstrated. This results in a 'shaggy' heart border with elevated diaphragms from progressive loss of lung volume.

Chronic cough, chest pain, haemoptysis and breathlessness 1

Radiological investigation

Carcinoma of the lung
- Chest X-ray (CXR)
- Computed tomography (CT) thorax and liver
- CT brain.

Lymphoma
- CXR
- CT thorax, abdomen, pelvis

Cryptogenic fibrosing alveolitis
- CXR
- High-resolution CT

Bronchiectasis
- CXR
- HRCT.

Chronic cough, chest pain, haemoptysis and breathlessness 2: tumours of the lung

Lung tumours can be conveniently divided into *primary* and *secondary* tumours.

Secondary lung tumours account for the large majority of neoplastic lesions within the lung. Box 1 lists the most common causative primary malignant lesions associated with metastatic disease in the lung.

Box 1 Primary tumours metastasizing to lung

- Kidney
- Breast
- Prostate
- Head and neck
- Thyroid.

Box 2 Carcinoma of the lung: cell types

- *Adenocarcinoma* (50%) – most common cell type in women and non smokers. These are usually peripherally located.
- *Squamous cell carcinoma* (30–35%) – strongly associated with cigarette smoking. Two-thirds are centrally located within the main, lobar or segmental bronchi.
- *Small cell carcinoma* (15%) – strongly associated with cigarette smoking. Rapid growth and high metastatic potential.
- *Large cell carcinoma* (<5%) – strongly associated with smoking. Usually peripherally located.

Radiological features

The typical plain chest film demonstrates multiple nodules of varying sizes (Fig. 1).

Primary lung tumours

Bronchogenic carcinoma
Carcinoma of the bronchus is the most common and important primary tumour of the lung and is the commonest fatal malignant tumour in adult males. Although it is more commonly seen in men, because of changes in social habit the increasing number of women smokers has given rise to an increased incidence of this tumour in females (Box 2). Carcinoma of the bronchus is rarely seen below the age of 30 and is most often seen between the ages of 50 and 70 years. The incidence of the tumour is related to the number of cigarettes smoked, whilst cessation of cigarette smoking diminishes the risk of the tumour. Smokers who also work with asbestos have an increased incidence of lung cancer and, similarly, those who work mining uranium or with nickel and arsenic have an increased incidence of lung cancer too.

Forty-two thousand new cases of lung cancer are diagnosed every year in the UK, accounting for 16% of all cancers diagnosed in males and 12% in females. The prognosis generally speaking is poor, with a 5-year survival rate of around 5%. Most cases of lung cancer are associated with cigarette smoking and since the pioneering work of Sir Richard Doll and Sir Richard Peto, the association between cigarette smoking and lung cancer has been recognized many times.

In the UK lung cancer deaths have approximately halved since 1965, but smoking is still the major cause of early death in the UK. Smoking does not merely cause lung cancer – it is also associated with coronary artery disease, chronic bronchitis and emphysema and cancers of the pancreas, and even bladder. Smoking pipes and aspirating tar are also associated with carcinoma of the mouth and oesophagus.

Clinical features

Fifty per cent of lung tumours arise centrally, that is, proximal to the segmental bronchi. The tumour, which arises in the mucosa of the bronchus grows into the bronchial lumen, obstructing it. The lung distal to the obstruction collapses. Air is resorbed and the lung then appears solid and consolidated. Infection arises distal to the obstruction.

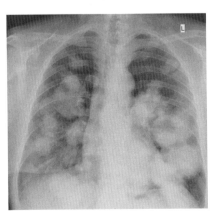

Fig. 1 **Metastatic disease in the lungs.** Multiple 'cannon ball' metastases are seen in both hemithoraces.

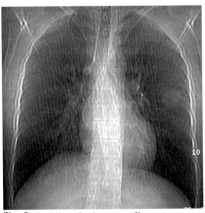

Fig. 2 **Peripheral primary malignant disease.** A scout view from a computed tomography scan demonstrating a lung mass in the left mid zone.

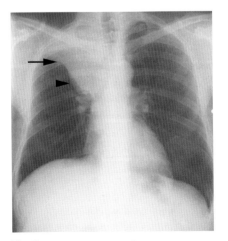

Fig. 3 **Central primary malignant tumour** (arrowhead). The 'S sign of Golden' – incomplete right upper lobar collapse and consolidation with a bulging contour produced by a primary tumour of the right hilum. Note the elevated horizontal fissure (arrow).

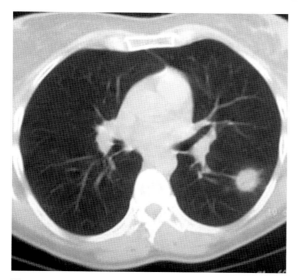

Fig. 4 **Peripheral primary malignant disease.** (Same patient as in Fig. 2.) A spiculated solid mass is shown in the apical segment of the left upper zone.

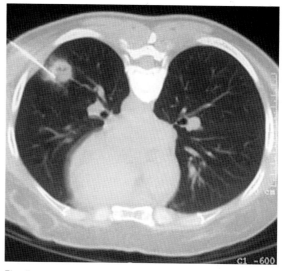

Fig. 5 **Peripheral primary malignant disease.** The patient is prone. A *Trucut* biopsy needle is seen in situ.

The symptoms of central tumours are cough, wheezing, haemoptysis, pneumonia and lung collapse.

Peripheral tumours are seen as round or spiculated nodules in the lung parenchyma. There may be collapse of lung distal to the tumour but this will be much smaller than if the obstructing tumour is centrally situated. Peripheral tumours may produce local chest pain or Pancoast syndrome. Superior vena cava obstruction (SVCO), in which occlusion of the superior vena cava causes distension of the veins in the head and neck, and hoarseness due to involvement of the recurrent laryngeal nerve, may be caused by more central tumours.

Oesophageal compression and invasion may result from a central malignant tumour or related mediastinal lymph nodes. The oesophagus may be compressed or invaded and the patient may present with dysphagia. Local invasion of the phrenic nerve may cause paralysis of the diaphragm, which will fail to move on a chest X-ray between expiration and inspiration.

Peripheral and central tumours may metastasize to the local hilar or mediastinal lymph nodes, which enlarge, again causing central bronchial obstruction.

Lung cancer metastasizes also to supraclavicular lymph nodes, as well as to the liver, the skeleton and the brain, the suprarenal glands and the skin.

Plain radiography

An ill-defined lung mass is the typical radiological finding on the chest film (Fig. 2). If the mass causes bronchial obstruction, collapse of one or more lobes of the lung may occur (Fig. 3).

Computed tomography

The role of cross-sectional imaging of the thorax and liver, as well as the brain, is to assess the local and distant spread of disease and to aid in histological diagnosis (Figs 4 & 5).

Tumours of the lung

- Tumours of the lung may be primary or secondary.
- Primary tumours are often related to cigarette smoking.
- On the chest film they are ill-defined with a spiculated margin (*corona maligna*).
- Benign tumours tend to be round, smooth and often calcified.
- Malignant tumours may be associated with dysphagia or peripheral lung collapse and infection.

Chronic cough, chest pain, haemoptysis and breathlessness 3: granulomatous lung disease

Tuberculosis

Tuberculosis (TB) causes more deaths in the world than any other infectious disease. In England and Wales during the period before and just after World War II there were around 50 000 cases each year, and it was a major cause of death – TB accounted for 6% of total human deaths in Britain in the 1930s and 1940s. There were numerous sanatoria in which patients were treated in the open air. TB was then acquired from drinking unpasteurized cows milk, and, until recently, there were still two or three deaths a year from TB acquired in this way, as this type of milk was still available in rural areas (green top milk). All milk is now pasteurized and, therefore, TB acquired from drinking contaminated milk no longer occurs. Since the advent of antibiotic treatment in 1948, the number of cases had fallen to around 5000 by the early 1990s. However, the numbers are rising, with around 7000 new cases being reported each year. Certain factors are responsible for the increase in the incidence of TB within particular groups (Box 1).

As can be seen from Box 2 the largest number of TB-related deaths in 2000 were seen in South and South East Asia. This has been associated

with large populations living closely together, resulting in the spread of TB within the family. The spread of HIV in drug addicts also accounts for an increase in incidence. The incidence of TB in Eastern Europe is interesting and probably related to poverty and families living in close proximity.

The radiological features of TB should be considered either as those related to the primary infection (**primary pulmonary** TB) or those features related to reactivation of the primary infection (**post-primary TB**).

Primary pulmonary tuberculosis

The mode of infection is inhalation of infected airborne droplets (Box 3). This

---

Box 1 Factors causing increased susceptibility to tuberculosis

- Growing poverty
- Homelessness
- Political instability and emigration
- Reductions in public healthcare provision
- Intravenous drug use
- HIV/AIDS infection
- New resistant strains of tuberculosis bacteria.

Box 2 Geographical incidence of tuberculosis in 2000

- South East Asia: 3 952 000
- Western Pacific: 2 255 000
- Africa: 2 079 000
- East Mediterranean: 870 000
- South America: 645 000
- Eastern Europe: 210 000
- Western Europe, USA, Canada, Australia, Japan and New Zealand: 211 000.

Box 3 Natural history of primary infection

- *Immunity* develops following primary infection.
- *Progressive primary tuberculosis (TB)* – this occurs in 10%, usually due to immune system deficiency.
- *Miliary TB* – secondary to uncontrolled massive haematogenous dissemination. Chest X-ray shows diffuse small nodules of pinpoint to 2–3 mm in size.
- *Post-primary TB* – reactivation after many years.

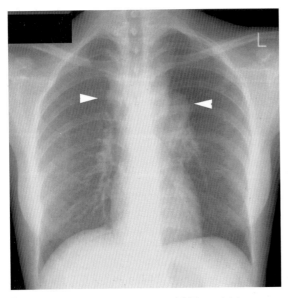

Fig. 1 **Primary tuberculosis.** Massive left hilar and right paratracheal adenopathy (arrows).

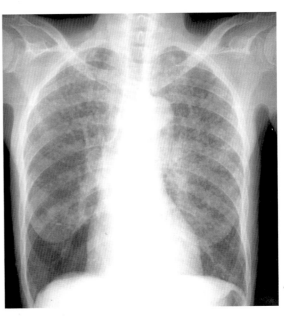

Fig. 2 **Miliary tuberculosis.** Generalized small nodules varying from pinpoint to 2–3 mm in size can be seen.

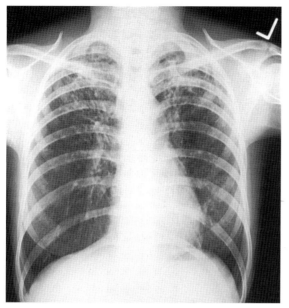

Fig. 3 **Post-primary tuberculosis.** Scarring, secondary to fibrosis, is seen extending into both upper lobes.

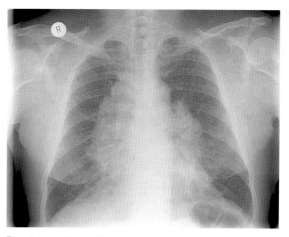

Fig. 4 **Sarcoidosis.** The '1–2–3 sign' – involvement of the right paratracheal and right and left hilar nodes.

usually occurs in childhood with most (90%) children asymptomatic.

Radiological features
There are ill-defined areas of airspace, segmental or lobar, consolidation, typically in the lower lobes, middle lobe or anterior segment of the upper. Massive hilar (60%), paratracheal (40%) and subcarinal adenopathy may occur in children (Fig. 1) (see Fig. 2 for miliary TB).

Post-primary pulmonary tuberculosis (reactivation tuberculosis)
The incidence of post-primary pulmonary TB is 1–10% per year, depending on the individual's immune system status.

Radiologically, this usually affects the apical and posterior segments of the upper lobes (85%) and superior segment of the lower lobes (10%). There is thick-walled irregular cavitation, with scarring (Fig. 3) and

bronchiectasis in the upper lobes. Calcified hilar and mediastinal nodes are seen.

Pleural effusion and empyema may develop, and the pleura may calcify in chronic disease, giving sheets of irregular calcification.

Colonization of the upper lobe cavities with *Aspergillus* may occur, forming an aspergilloma (or fungus ball) (see Box 4 for a list of tuberculosis-causing organisms).

Sarcoidosis

Sarcoidosis is a widespread multisystem granulomatous condition of unknown aetiology. It presents most frequently in black females (M:F = 1:3; blacks:Caucasians = 14:1). Thoracic disease occurs in 90% of patients with angiotensin-converting enzyme (ACE) elevated in 70%.

In its acute form, patients present with *bilateral hilar adenopathy*, fever, erythema nodosum and arthralgia. In

the chronic form of the disease 50% of patients are asymptomatic, but progressive shortness of breath (25%) and haemoptysis (4%) are frequent presenting complaints.

Radiological features
The most common radiological finding is that of hilar lymphadenopathy, which is seen in about 80% of cases. The involvement also of the right paratracheal nodes gives a characteristic '1–2–3 sign' (Fig. 4).

Over time, involved lymph nodes may calcify, sometimes with egg-shell calcification at the margin of the nodes.

Interstitial fibrosis is also seen sometimes with the formation of large air spaces in the lungs. This occurs in up to 60% of patients, giving a reticulonodular pattern. Progressive disease gives an appearance not unlike that in TB, but there are no calcifying granulomas in the periphery of the lungs.

Box 4 Organisms causing tuberculosis

Mycobacterium tuberculosis (95%)
Atypical mycobacteria are on the increase:
- *M. avium-intracellulare*
- *M. kansasii*
- *M. fortuitum*.

Granulomatous lung disease

- Tuberculosis may be primary or post-primary.
- It is of increased incidence in deprived sections of the community.
- It is becoming a major health problem.
- Sarcoid is an uncommon condition, but has characteristic radiological features of hilar adenopathy going on to fibrosis.

Chronic cough, chest pain, haemoptysis and breathlessness 4: bronchiectasis and cystic fibrosis

Bronchiectasis

Bronchiectasis is the term used to describe irreversible bronchial dilatation. Box 1 lists the different aetiologies for bronchiectasis.

Patients with interstitial fibrosis have a distortion of the lung anatomy and their bronchi become dilated (traction bronchiectasis). Cylindrical or tubular bronchiectasis results in a dilated bronchus with parallel walls (Box 2). Saccular bronchiectasis shows dilated saccules at the ends of the bronchi. In varicose bronchiectasis there is more irregular dilatation of the bronchi.

Box 1 Aetiology of bronchiectasis

Congenital
- Abnormal mucociliary transport: *Kartagener's syndrome*
- Abnormal secretions: mucoviscidosis (*cystic fibrosis*)
- Immune deficiency: IgG deficiency.

Acquired
- Post-infectious: measles, whooping cough, tuberculosis
- Bronchial obstruction
- Aspiration.

No cause for bronchiectasis is found in over 50% of cases.

Box 2 Classification of bronchiectasis

- Cylindrical/tubular bronchiectasis
- Saccular/cystic bronchiectasis
- Varicose bronchiectasis (rare).

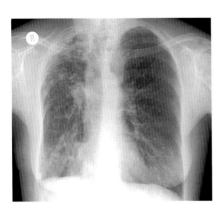

Fig. 1 **Bronchiectasis.** Marked bronchial wall thickening in the right lower lobe with associated 'tram line' formation. Note old fibrosis and volume loss in the right upper lobe secondary to previous tuberculosis.

Plain radiography

On the plain chest film the lower lobes of the chest are mainly affected (Fig. 1) with an increase in the size of the lung markings due to retained secretions. Bronchial wall thickening is seen, together with cystic air spaces and 'tram-lines' with or without air-fluid levels in dilated bronchi. Tram-lines represent thick-walled, dilated bronchi.

Computed tomography

High-resolution CT (HRCT) scanning shows lack of tapering of bronchi (Fig. 2). The most obvious findings are 'tram lines', which are seen with bronchi orientated horizontally to the plain film or CT scan. The 'signet-ring sign' is seen with bronchi perpendicular to the scan plane – a cross-section of dilated bronchus is larger than that of the accompanying branch of pulmonary artery (Fig. 3). Cystic dilatation of the bronchi towards the periphery of the lung is seen in severe cases.

Cystic fibrosis

In this multisystem disease a defective gene causes an abnormality of mucus and sweat secretion. In the respiratory system the mucus formed is thick and viscid, which blocks the airways and causes changes of distal infection, bronchiectasis and fibrosis (Fig. 4). Gastrointestinal absorption is also hindered due to an abnormal pancreas, while male infertility also results.

Radiologically, the changes are those of bronchial wall thickening and

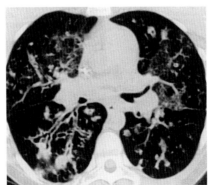

Fig. 2 **Cylindrical or tubular bronchiectasis.** Computed tomography at the level of the hila demonstrates widespread bronchiectasis (well seen in the apical segment of the right upper lobe). The bronchi fail to taper and have irregular thickened walls. (Reproduced with permission from Sutton (ed.) *Textbook of radiology and imaging*, 7th edn. Churchill Livingstone, Edinburgh, 2002.)

bronchiectasis, together with prominent hilar shadows. The hilar enlargement is due to enlarged lymph nodes caused by chronic infection, and enlargement of the central pulmonary arteries is due to pulmonary artery hypertension. These changes are best assessed using HRCT.

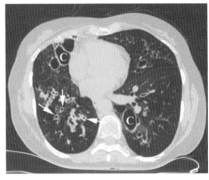

Fig. 3 **Bronchiectasis** – HRCT. Widespread cystic dilatation of the bronchi (C), predominantly in the right middle and left lower lobes. The dilated bronchus contains air and shows as black, whereas the pulmonary artery contains blood and is solid, and therefore opaque (white) to the X-ray beam (arrow). Note the marked bronchial wall thickening and several 'signet rings' (arrowheads) in the right lower lobe.

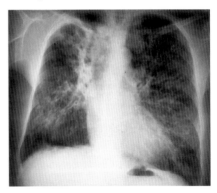

Fig. 4 **Cystic fibrosis.** The lungs are hyperinflated. Thickened walls of dilated bronchi seen in both lungs, producing densities that resemble tramlines. Branching, band-like shadows in the left lower zone are caused by dilated bronchi filled with secretions. (Courtesy of Dr J. Batten, Brompton Hospital)

Bronchiectasis and cystic fibrosis

- Bronchiectasis follows childhood infection or adult tuberculosis or aspiration.
- Bronchiectasis may result in repeated chest infections.
- Cystic fibrosis is the result of a faulty gene and thickened secretions. In the chest this results in bronchiectasis, fibrotic changes and repeated chest infections.
- With modern treatments many patients with cystic fibrosis are living into adult life.

Gastrointestinal System

Radiological techniques and the gastrointestinal tract

Practically every form of medical imaging has a role in the investigation of the gastrointestinal tract. The choice of investigation is largely dependent on the clinical question posed and will be described in the later chapters. In essence, however, the gastrointestinal tract essentially comprises a long tube with various solid appendages (the liver and pancreas for example) and a broad distinction may be drawn between those imaging techniques that best visualize the tube (e.g. barium studies), and those that best visualize the organs (e.g. ultrasound, computed tomography). The following gives an overview of the techniques most commonly used by the radiologist in day-to-day clinical practice.

Plain radiography

The plain abdominal X-ray is frequently performed, although very few disease processes give specific plain film findings. It is mainly requested to look at the bowel gas pattern (distribution of gas throughout the gastrointestinal tract) and is, therefore, most useful for diagnosis of bowel obstruction. Viscus perforation may also be manifest by free intra-abdominal gas.

Contrast studies

Barium examinations

Barium sulphate suspension is a high-density liquid that is easily visualized due to its ability to absorb X-rays. The oesophagus, stomach, small bowel and colon can all be imaged when their lumen is filled or coated by barium suspension, but the precise technique used varies widely depending on the organ under investigation. Studies can be performed with barium alone ('single contrast'), or with additional gaseous distension of the bowel such that barium forms a thin coating on the mucosa ('double contrast') (Fig. 1).

Video endoscopy has largely replaced barium studies of the oesophagus and stomach due to its higher sensitivity for mucosal lesions and an ability to take biopsies. However, the barium swallow

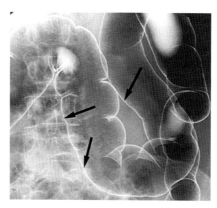

Fig. 1 **Normal barium enema.** Note that the colon has been distended with gas so that the barium forms a thin line (arrows) coating the mucosal surface and giving a double contrast effect.

(oesophagus) and barium meal (stomach) are still performed in patients intolerant of endoscopy or those with suspected motility disorders. In both examinations patients drink barium suspension. In the case of the barium meal, the patient swallows an effervescent agent to distend the stomach with carbon dioxide gas, facilitating double contrast views. Barium examination still forms the mainstay of small bowel investigation due to its relative inaccessibility to endoscopy. Separation of small bowel loops by compression during fluoroscopic X-ray screening aids diagnosis (Fig. 2).

The barium enema is widely performed due to its reasonable sensitivity for colonic pathology,

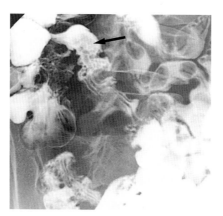

Fig. 2 **Compression view from a barium follow through study** shows a normal terminal ileum (arrow).

including cancer and diverticular disease, although it may be difficult in very elderly or immobile patients. A double contrast technique is preferred, gas being introduced into the colon via a rectal tube.

Non-barium contrast studies

Barium is highly irritant if spilled in the peritoneal cavity or mediastinum, causing an intense fibrotic reaction, which may prove fatal. Water-soluble contrast (either ionic or non-ionic) should, therefore, be used if there is a possibility of intestinal perforation or if there is a recent surgical anastamosis. Such contrast can be administered orally or per rectum and is mainly used in cases of bowel obstruction or if the integrity of a surgical anastamosis is questioned.

Cross-sectional imaging

Ultrasound

Ultrasound is a technique whereby high-frequency sound pulses are emitted into the tissue of interest and an image formed based on the characteristics of the reflected energies. The major advantages of ultrasound are that it is quick, cheap, and safe but it is operator dependent. Fat, gas and bone all attenuate sound, and so deep structures within the abdominal cavity, such as the pancreas, are often poorly seen. However, the technique is very good at examining solid organs, particularly the liver (Fig. 3), gall bladder, spleen and kidneys, and is often the first-line imaging investigation when pathology is suspected.

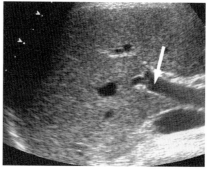

Fig. 3 **Ultrasound image of a normal liver.** Note the portal vein (arrow).

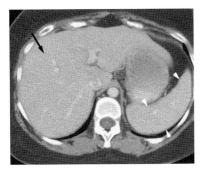

Fig. 4 **Contrast-enhanced CT scan through the upper abdomen** showing a normal liver (arrow) and spleen (arrowheads).

Computed tomography

Computed tomography (CT) scanners emit a thin X-ray beam from an X-ray tube that rotates around the patient, and gives multiple axial slices for analysis (Fig. 4). Most CT scans are performed with intravenous iodine contrast to enhance lesion identification, although care must be taken in those with allergic conditions, such as asthma and those with impaired renal function. In comparison to ultrasound, CT is relatively expensive and carries theoretical risks associated with the relatively large radiation dose, particularly in younger patients. However, it is generally more sensitive than ultrasound and provides information from the whole abdominal cavity. It is routinely used in abdominal trauma, investigation of abdominal pain, suspected abdominal malignancy or abscesses, and for further characterization of lesions detected with ultrasound. Good information regarding the small and large bowel is also obtained, particularly the extramural extent of disease.

Magnetic resonance imaging

Magnetic resonance imaging (MRI) has many of the advantages of CT, but, importantly, it is not ionizing radiation that is used, but the differences in the magnetic properties of body tissues, and these are used to construct the image.

MRI is particularly good at imaging fluid, which appears white on certain images sequences. This property is utilized in obtaining exquisite images of the biliary tree, and for the detection of small tracts and sinuses arising from bowel. Due to limitation in access to MRI technology, the technique is currently mainly used for lesion detection, characterization in the liver and pancreas, imaging the biliary tree and characterizing perianal fistulae, but there are many other potential uses in the abdomen.

Interventional imaging

Either CT or ultrasound guides many interventional procedures within the abdomen, such as biopsy or abscess drainage. Angiographic techniques are also used within the abdomen, most commonly to diagnose and treat acute intestinal haemorrhage.

Endoscopic retrograde cholangiopancreatography and percutaneous transhepatic cholangiography

Imaging and intervention within the biliary tree, however, often requires endoscopic retrograde cholangiopancreatography (ERCP). A specialized endoscope is used to enable the operator to access the ampulla of Vater in the duodenum in order to inject contrast medium to outline the biliary tree or pancreatic duct. Percutaneous transhepatic cholangiography (PTC) is reserved for those patients intolerant of endoscopy or in whom access through the ampulla is not possible, for example, due to obstructing tumour. A needle is guided though the skin into the liver, and thence into the bile ducts, often under ultrasound guidance. Contrast medium is then injected to image the whole biliary tree. Both ERCP and PTC enable the deployment of stents to relieve biliary obstruction.

Nuclear medicine

Various nuclear medicine techniques find use within the abdomen, most notably white cell scans for the detection of occult infection, red cell scans for diagnosis of intestinal bleeding, and positron emission tomography (PET) scanning in the diagnosis and staging of intra-abdominal malignancy.

Radiological techniques and the gastrointestinal tract

- All imaging modalities have use in the gastrointestinal tract. The examination chosen is dependent on the clinical scenario.
- Contrast studies remain the mainstay of diagnosis within the small bowel, and remain useful in investigation of the stomach and colon.
- Ultrasound is quick and safe, and gives good information regarding solid organs.
- Computed tomography and magnetic resonance imaging are generally more sensitive than ultrasound and give information from the whole abdominal cavity.
- Interventional procedures such as endoscopic retrograde cholangiopancreatography and percutaneous transhepatic cholangiography are used for the diagnosis and treatment of disorders of the biliary tree.

Dysphagia

Dysphagia is defined as difficulty in swallowing food and/or liquid. It is a potentially serious symptom and usually merits further investigation. There are many causes of dysphagia, some of which are shown in Table 1.

Table 1 **Causes of dysphagia**		
Malignancy	**Benign disease**	**Motility disorders**
Pharyngeal cancer	Peptic stricture	Achalasia
Oesophageal cancer	Oesophageal webs	Bulbar palsy
Gastric cancer	Radiation/caustic stricture	Myasthenia gravis
Extrinsic compression, e.g. lung cancer	Pharyngeal pouch	Presbyoesophagus
	Systemic sclerosis (scleroderma)	Diffuse oesophageal spasm
	Foreign body	

Investigation of dysphagia

The nature of dysphagia may give clues to the underlying aetiology. For example, greater difficulty in swallowing liquids than solids suggests an underlying motility disorder, whereas a neck bulge with gurgling may suggest a pharyngeal pouch (herniation of mucosa through a weakness in the muscles of the pharynx) (Fig. 1). Weight loss and rapidly progressive dysphagia suggest underlying malignancy and warrant urgent investigation.

Dysphagia is usually investigated by means of fibre-optic endoscopy or barium swallow. Endoscopy has the advantage of giving exquisite views of the oesophageal mucosa and allows biopsy and interventional procedures

such as dilatation of strictures and stenting of tumours. However, it often requires intravenous sedation, which is potentially hazardous, particularly in the elderly or in those with pre-existing cardiorespiratory disorders.

The barium swallow is a safe and well-tolerated alternative and, although mucosal detail is less well seen than at endoscopy, it is able to demonstrate the majority of structural causes of dysphagia. Furthermore, it gives superior information regarding oesophageal configuration and function and is, therefore, the investigation of choice for suspected motility disorders as well as for those patients who may not tolerate endoscopy. A video recording of the barium swallow can be made to allow detailed step-by-step

analysis of the swallowing mechanism in patients with neurological disorders, for example after a stroke.

Carcinoma of the oesophagus

Carcinoma of the oesophagus most commonly presents with progressive dysphagia. Up to 60% of tumours are of the squamous cell type and are associated with smoking and high alcohol intake. There is an increased incidence in China, South Africa and in some parts of the Middle East, which may be due to dietary factors. Adenocarcinoma makes up the majority of the remaining cancers and is usually caused by dysplastic change in the lower oesophageal epithelium as a result of longstanding reflux oesophagitis (Barrett's oesophagus).

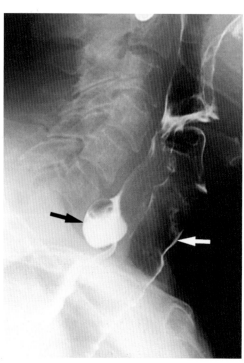

Fig. 1 **Barium swallow demonstrates a large pharyngeal pouch** (black arrow). Note the aspiration of contrast into the trachea (white arrow).

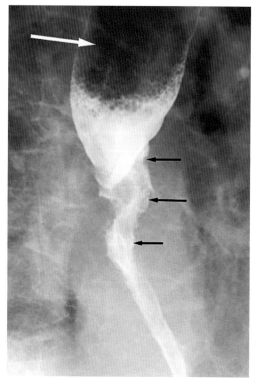

Fig. 2 **Barium swallow demonstrates an irregular stricture** in the mid oesophagus (black arrows) due to carcinoma. Note the dilated oesophagus (white arrow) above the stricture.

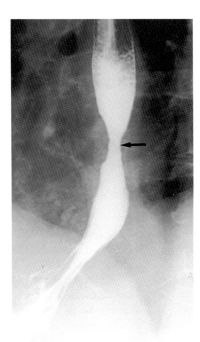

Fig. 3 **Barium swallow demonstrates a smooth peptic stricture** (arrow) just above the gastro-oesophageal junction.

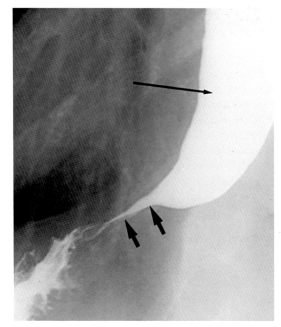

Fig. 4 **Barium swallow demonstrates the typical features of achalasia with dilated oesophagus** (long arrow) above an intermittently opening tapered gastro-oesophageal junction (short arrows), giving a 'rat's tail' appearance.

Cancer of the oesophagus usually appears as an irregular shouldered stricture on barium swallow (Fig. 2). Unfortunately, most tumours are advanced at the time of presentation, with spread to regional lymph nodes, and staging of these advanced tumours is best done with computed tomography (CT). Early cancers, that is those confined to the oesophageal wall, are best staged with endoscopic ultrasound, which shows the individual layers of the wall of the oesophagus.

Reflux and peptic stricture

Benign strictures of the oesophagus are usually the result of chronic reflux oesophagitis (peptic stricture). Although gastro-oesophageal reflux can be a normal finding, prolonged exposure of the oesophageal mucosa to acid and pepsin from the stomach can cause inflammation. Those with disordered motility, such as the elderly, or those with scleroderma, are particularly at risk because the oesophagus fails to clear the refluxed gastric contents.

There is an association between hiatus hernia of the stomach and reflux, although one can occur without the other. A hiatus hernia is usually well demonstrated during a barium swallow, although reflux is often intermittent and failure to demonstrate it during the study does not exclude the diagnosis.

The earliest changes of reflux oesophagitis are best seen at endoscopy, although as the disease progresses, mucosal nodularity and ulceration can be seen on barium swallow. Chronic scarring may lead to stricture formation, which is usually short and tapering on barium swallow (Fig. 3). Mucosal ulceration and oedema can also result in peptic strictures that mimic malignancy on barium swallow and endoscopy with biopsy is often necessary to distinguish between the two.

Motility disorders

Abnormal oesophageal motility is common with increasing age and occasionally may be so severe as to cause symptoms (presbyoesophagus). Barium swallow is able to demonstrate the abnormal oesophageal contractions, often combined with a failure of relaxation of the lower oesophageal sphincter.

Achalasia is a motility disorder characterized by failure of the lower oesophageal sphincter to relax and generally occurs in patients aged between 35 and 50 years. It is caused by degeneration of neurons in Auerbach's plexus and leads to disordered oesophageal contractions, eventually leading to a dilated oesophagus filled with food debris. Barium swallow demonstrates a baggy oesophagus with an intermittently opening tapered gastro-oesophageal junction, giving a 'rat's tail' appearance (Fig. 4). Treatment is usually by intermittent balloon dilatation of the lower sphincter during endoscopy.

Dysphagia

- Dysphagia may be a serious symptom and should be investigated.
- Endoscopy gives the best mucosal detail and allows biopsy, but is invasive.
- Barium swallow is safe and superior for diagnosis of motility disorders.
- Cancer of the oesophagus has a poor prognosis and is best staged with computed tomography.
- Apparently benign strictures on barium swallow often need confirmatory biopsy.
- Achalasia gives a characteristic rat's tail appearance on barium swallow.

Imaging liver disease

Patients with liver disease may present in several ways. They may have hepatomegaly or a liver mass, or demonstrate the stigmata of chronic liver disease such as jaundice, spider naevi, gynaecomastia, etc. Commonly, they are identified as a result of abnormal liver function tests or during the process of staging underlying neoplasia.

Whatever the presentation, imaging has a significant role in the investigation of the patient with suspected liver disease. The imaging techniques available are complementary, each having specific advantages and disadvantages and, in addition to giving structural information, imaging can guide therapeutic or diagnostic intervention.

Ultrasound is often the quickest, simplest and cheapest test to perform. It gives information regarding the size and texture of the liver, detects focal abnormality, and accurately assesses the biliary tree. It is often used for image-guided liver intervention, particularly liver biopsy of focal lesions. The sensitivity of ultrasound is, however, highly operator dependent and there are particular difficulties when examining obese patients, as adipose tissue significantly attenuates the ultrasound beam. To ensure the liver is fully examined with ultrasound, patients often are required to turn onto their side and so there may be problems examining very immobile patients.

Computed tomography (CT) of the liver, performed with intravenous iodinated contrast medium, is excellent for the detection and characterization of focal liver lesions, and is often used to monitor treatment in patients with hepatic metastasis. It also gives information about the hepatic arterial and portal venous systems, and can obviate the need for more interventional tests such as angiography. CT is less operator dependent than ultrasound, but is more expensive and exposes the patient to a significant radiation dose.

Magnetic resonance imaging (MRI) of the liver is usually reserved for problem solving, particularly for the characterization of liver lesions. It does not utilize ionizing radiation, but is complex and relatively time consuming compared with CT and ultrasound.

Diffuse liver disease and cirrhosis

The major role of imaging in patients with abnormal liver function tests is to exclude focal liver lesions or structural abnormalities such as biliary dilatation. There are many causes of hepatitis, very few of which give specific diagnostic features on any imaging modality. All may cause change in liver echogenicity on ultrasound but, ultimately, diagnosis relies on history, serology and biopsy.

Common causes of liver cirrhosis include alcohol and post viral hepatitis, with rarer causes including Wilson's disease and haemochromatosis. The changes in cirrhosis are similar on all imaging modalities and include a shrunken, irregular and nodular liver (Fig. 1). Portal hypertension is a common sequela of cirrhosis and an enlarged portal vein with abnormal Doppler trace is seen on ultrasound, along with coexistent varices, splenomegaly and ascites.

Patients with cirrhosis are at risk of developing hepatocellular carcinoma, which should be suspected in patients with increasing right upper quadrant pain and rising serum alpha–feto protein. The coarse liver echogenicity on ultrasound may make it difficult to detect small tumours and if clinical suspicion is high, CT or MRI is more sensitive.

Focal liver lesions

There are many causes of focal liver lesions as outlined in Table 1.

Ultrasound is the best initial investigation in patients suspected of having a focal liver abnormality, for example liver metastasis. While ultrasound will detect most significant liver lesions, it will miss a small, but significant, minority of focal abnormalities, usually because the lesion appears very similar to the normal surrounding liver or because the patient is difficult to examine.

The most common focal liver abnormality is a simple cyst, which is confidently diagnosed with ultrasound without the need for any further tests (Fig. 2). Benign hepatic haemangiomas also have characteristic appearances on ultrasound, typically being very echogenic, well-defined lesions, and further imaging can be reserved for only those lesions with atypical appearances.

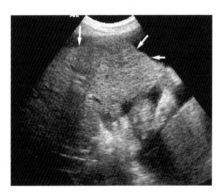

Fig. 1 **Ultrasound of the liver** demonstrates an irregular border (arrows) due to cirrhosis.

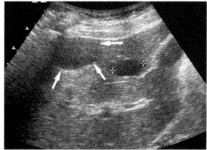

Fig. 2 **Ultrasound of the liver** shows a well defined anechoic lesion (crosses) characteristic of a simple cyst. A second larger cyst (arrows) is also seen.

Table 1 **Causes of focal liver lesions**		
Malignant	**Benign**	**Infective**
Primary hepatocellular carcinoma	Simple cyst	Pyogenic liver abscess
Metastases	Haemangioma	Amoebic abscess
Lymphoma/Leukaemia	Adenoma	Hydatid disease
Biliary tumours	Focal nodular hyperplasia	Tuberculosis

Many other causes of focal liver abnormalities have similar appearances on ultrasound but, when put in the context of the clinical presentation, further investigations may not be required to manage the patient. For example, a patient with known malignancy and multiple focal lesions on ultrasound is highly likely to have liver metastases, while a low echogenicity lesion in a patient with a swinging fever, leukocytosis and right upper-quadrant pain is almost certainly a liver abscess.

Many causes of focal liver lesions have characteristic features on contrast-enhanced CT, for example haemangiomas (Fig. 3) and metastases (Fig. 4), and CT is, therefore, used for lesion identification. In many cases this avoids the need for invasive biopsy. CT will often detect lesions missed with ultrasound, and is the preferred modality to follow-up patients with liver metastases who are undergoing therapy.

MRI is superior to CT for characterizing liver lesions, particularly when trying to differentiate between benign and malignant disease processes. The technique is, therefore, reserved for problem solving when CT and ultrasound have not given the answer.

The use of imaging for the investigation of liver disease is outlined in Figure 5.

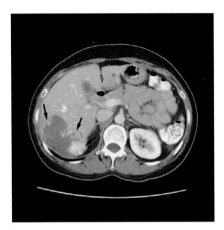

Fig. 3 **Computed tomography scan through the liver** demonstrates peripheral pooling of intravenous contrast medium (arrows) around a low attenuation lesion, typical of a haemangioma.

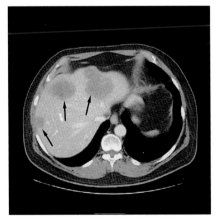

Fig. 4 **Contrast enhanced computed tomography scan of the liver** shows multiple irregular low attenuation lesions (arrows) due to metastases.

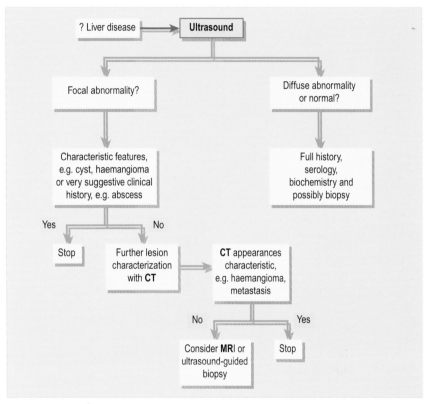

Fig. 5 **Flowchart of imaging techniques for the investigation of liver disease.**

Imaging liver disease

- Ultrasound is the first-line radiological investigation in suspected liver disease.

- Liver cirrhosis commonly leads to a shrunken irregular liver with splenomegaly and ascites.

- Computed tomography (CT) or magnetic resonance imaging (MRI) are more sensitive than ultrasound in detecting hepatocellular carcinoma in patients with cirrhosis.

- In the context of the clinical presentation, ultrasound may be sufficient to manage a patient with a focal liver lesion.

- Both CT and MRI are superior to ultrasound, both in lesion detection and in characterization.

Disorders of the gallbladder and biliary tree

Gall bladder and biliary tree

Anatomy

Bile drains from hepatocytes into a canalicular network of tiny ducts that run with the portal vein and hepatic artery in the portal triad. The interlobular ducts unite to form septal bile ducts, which themselves unite to form the left and right main hepatic ducts. The two main hepatic ducts fuse at the liver hilum to form the common hepatic duct, which runs in the free edge of the lesser omentum. It is joined by the cystic duct from the gall bladder and thereafter becomes the common bile duct, finally inserting via the ampulla of Vater into the second part of the duodenum.

Gallbladder

Most gallbladder pathology in adults is secondary to gallstones. Gallstones are common and occur in 10% of adults over the age of 50 years in developed countries, being much less common in the third world. Factors associated with an increased risk of gallstones include female sex, obesity, haemolytic disorders and diseases of the terminal ileum (where bile salts are normally reabsorbed).

Eighty per cent of gallstones are asymptomatic. Most symptomatic patients experienced biliary colic. While colic may be transient, impaction of a stone in the gallbladder neck or cystic duct can lead to gallbladder inflammation and acute cholecystitis, which may become chronic after repeated attacks. Rarely, an empyema of the gall bladder due to the stagnant infected bile may occur, and is a serious condition requiring drainage.

If stones become impacted in the common bile duct, they may cause acute pancreatitis (see p. 62) or obstructive jaundice (see p. 60).

Gallbladder carcinoma is a relatively rare tumour and when it occurs, is usually in the presence of gallstones. The tumour is often clinically silent, presenting at an advanced stage.

Imaging the gallbladder

Ultrasound is the imaging investigation of choice for suspected gallbladder pathology. Patients must be

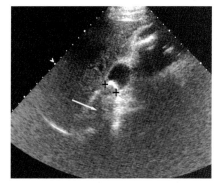

Fig. 1 **Ultrasound of the gallbladder shows the typical appearance of a gallstone** (crosses). Note the distal acoustic shadow (arrow) due to non-transmission of sound waves through the stone.

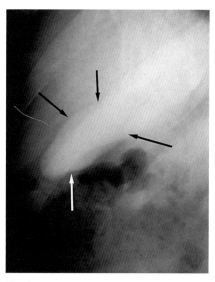

Fig. 2 **X-ray performed during an oral cholecystogram** demonstrates contrast medium within the gallbladder (arrows), indicating normal function.

starved before the scan to ensure the gallbladder is optimally distended with bile. Gallstones are seen as bright objects within the gallbladder lumen, classically producing an acoustic 'shadow' due to the non-transmission of sound by calcium within the stones (Fig. 1).

Acute cholecystitis produces a distended, thick-walled, tender gallbladder on ultrasound, often with a rim of surrounding fluid. In chronic cholecystitis the gallbladder is thick walled but contracted. Such is the accuracy of ultrasound, that other imaging techniques, such as oral cholecystography (Fig. 2) in which a patient swallows iodinated compounds excreted by the gall bladder, are reserved for investigation of gallbladder function rather than structure.

Biliary tree

Congenital disorders of the biliary tree are rare and often present in the first few weeks of life. Cystic dilatation of the common bile duct (choledochal cyst) may, however, present later with jaundice and abdominal pain, and should be considered in any young

patient presenting with symptoms of biliary disease. The most common disorder of the biliary tree is impaction of gallstones within the ducts. However, biliary strictures, both benign and malignant, are not uncommon (Table 1).

Primary sclerosing cholangitis (Fig. 3) is characterized by an inflammatory process affecting the intra- and extrahepatic bile ducts. It may present with symptoms of biliary obstruction at any age and is associated with inflammatory bowel disease (especially ulcerative colitis) and autoimmune disorders. Patients have an increased risk of developing cholangiocarcinoma (bile duct tumour).

Imaging the biliary tree

Ultrasound is very sensitive at detecting biliary dilatation (see p. 60) and may also identify the underlying cause, for example by demonstrating a pancreatic mass or local compressing lymphadenopathy. It has relatively low

Table 1 **Causes of biliary stricture**	
Benign	**Malignant**
Post surgical, e.g. cholecystectomy, liver transplant	Cholangiocarcinoma
Trauma	Ampullary and pancreatic carcinoma
Primary sclerosing cholangitis	Invasion by local malignant spread
AIDS cholangiopathy	
Chronic pancreatitis	
Parasitic infections	

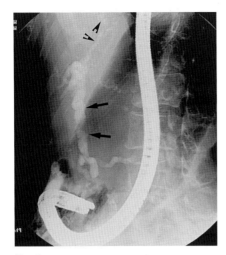

Fig. 3 **Endoscopic retrograde cholangiopancreatography** shows irregularity of the common bile duct (arrows) and intrahepatic ducts (arrowheads) in keeping with sclerosing cholangitis.

Table 2 **Comparison of ERCP, MRCP and PTC**			
Feature	ERCP	PTC	MRCP
Invasive	++	+	–
Allow biopsy	++	+/–	–
Complications, e.g. pancreatitis, bleeding	++	+	–
Allows intervention, e.g. stent deployment	++	–	–
Visualizes pancreatic duct	++	–	+

sensitivity in detecting bile duct stones due to the duct being obscured by gas in the adjacent duodenum. It is also poor at demonstrating intrinsic bile-duct pathology such as strictures.

Contrast studies are the imaging investigation of choice for demonstrating bile duct strictures. Two techniques are available: endoscopic retrograde cholangiopancreatography (ERCP) and percutaneous transhepatic cholangiography (PTC).

Both techniques involve cannulation of the biliary tree followed by injection of contrast medium under X-ray control. In ERCP the biliary tree is accessed by the intubation of the ampulla of Vater using a specially designed endoscope. During PTC a needle is passed percutaneously through the liver under X-ray and/or ultrasound control into a peripheral intrahepatic duct to access the biliary tree.

In recent years a non-invasive method of imaging the biliary tree has been devised using magnetic resonance imaging (MRI) called magnetic resonance cholangiopancreatography (MRCP). A special MRI sequence is used such that fluid in the biliary tree and pancreatic duct is highlighted so that the ducts can be easily visualized. The technique is safe and non-invasive and can demonstrate bile duct stones (Fig. 4) and strictures with accuracies approaching ERCP, and has the benefit of giving additional information regarding tumour stage in malignant strictures. A comparison of the features of ERCP, MRCP and PTC is shown in Table 2.

The role of these techniques in the investigation and treatment of biliary obstruction is given on pages 60–61.

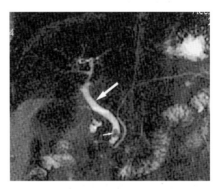

Fig. 4 **Coronal image from a magnetic resonance cholangiopancreatography examination** demonstrates a stone (small arrow) in the fluid-filled common bile duct (long arrow).

Disorders of the gallbladder and biliary tree

- Most clinical problems related to the gall bladder are due to gallstones, although most are asymptomatic.
- Ultrasound is the imaging investigation of choice for the gallbladder and biliary tree.
- Endoscopic retrograde cholangiopancreatography (ERCP) or percutaneous transhepatic cholangiography (PTC) are the preferred examinations for demonstrating biliary strictures.
- Magnetic resonance cholangiopancreatography is a non-invasive technique of imaging the biliary tree, giving diagnostic accuracies similar to ERCP and PTC.

Obstructive jaundice

Jaundice refers to yellow skin and mucous membranes due to a raised plasma bilirubin (usually >35 µmol/L). Bilirubin is formed by the breakdown of haemoglobin and is conjugated in the liver before being excreted in the bile.

Causes of jaundice can be divided into pre-hepatic causes such as haemolysis, hepatocellular causes such as hepatitis or drugs, and causes of obstruction to the excretion of bile. A full history and examination with appropriate blood tests are essential in all patients presenting with jaundice.

Bilirubin is converted by intestinal bacteria into stercobilinogen, which gives faeces their brown colour. Unconjugated bilirubin is insoluble, whereas conjugated bilirubin is water soluble and appears in the urine when present in excess in the blood stream. The presence, therefore, of dark urine and pale stools in a jaundiced patient suggests obstruction to the excretion of bile from the liver into the intestine. The most common underlying causes are shown in Box 1.

Imaging the jaundiced patient

The initial role of imaging in the jaundiced patient is to establish whether there is dilatation of the biliary tree, which suggests obstruction as the cause.

Ultrasound is the initial imaging modality of choice to evaluate the biliary tree. The common hepatic duct is well seen above the portal vein at the liver hilum and accurate measurement of its diameter can be made. It is dilated when it measures over 10 mm (less in young patients) (Fig. 1).

In addition to examining the extrahepatic biliary tree, ultrasound can demonstrate dilatation of the intrahepatic ducts running within the liver parenchyma. In the absence of biliary dilatation it is unlikely (although not impossible) that jaundice is due to obstruction.

Because both the common bile duct and pancreas may be obscured by gas within the stomach and duodenum, ultrasound may not demonstrate the cause of the obstruction. It is particularly poor at demonstrating stones within the common bile duct.

Identifying the cause of jaundice

After the initial ultrasound, the next imaging method, if any, depends both on the scan findings and the clinical presentation. The presence of sudden-onset pain with relatively acute jaundice in an otherwise well patient suggests an underlying impacted gallstone, whereas progressive painless jaundice in an unwell patient is more suspicious of underlying malignancy. Constitutional symptoms suggest hepatitis.

If the symptoms/ultrasound suggest gallstones, then endoscopic retrograde cholangiopancreatography (ERCP) is both diagnostic and enables therapeutic manoeuvres to remove the duct stones (Fig. 2). Magnetic resonance cholangiopancreatography (MRCP) can also be performed in patients in whom ERCP is dangerous or not possible. Both ERCP and MRCP are described on pages 58–59.

If the findings are more suggestive of an underlying malignant process, then computed tomography (CT) or magnetic resonance imaging (MRI) is indicated to demonstrate any pancreatic mass, features of chronic pancreatitis or compressing lymph nodes, etc. Both imaging modalities give information regarding the operability of any tumour and allow planning of therapy.

Relief of jaundice

The treatment of patients with obstructive jaundice has been revolutionized by the introduction of biliary stents. These stents are placed in the common bile duct across the cause of the obstruction in order to allow free passage of bile (Fig. 3).

Both ERCP and percutaneous transhepatic cholangiography (PTC) can be used to place biliary stents. PTC is particularly useful in those patients in whom it is difficult or impossible to perform ERCP, for example those with large tumours, previous gastric surgery, or intolerant of endoscopy.

Box 1 Causes of extrahepatic obstructive jaundice

- Gallstones
- Bile duct strictures: benign and malignant
- Chronic pancreatitis
- Pancreatic carcinoma
- Extrinsic compression of the bile duct, e.g. by enlarged lymph nodes.

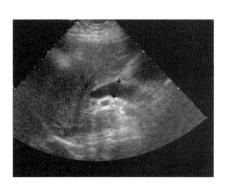

Fig. 1 **Ultrasound of the liver** demonstrates a dilated common bile duct (crosses).

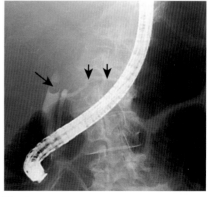

Fig. 2 **Endoscopic retrograde cholangio-pancreatography** demonstrates a stone (long arrow) in the common bile duct. Note contrast medium also fills the pancreatic duct (short arrows).

In general, biliary stenting is performed for palliation in patients with inoperable malignancy, but it also has a role in providing temporary relief of jaundice before more definitive treatment such as surgery for operable malignancies, or repeat ERCP for removal of impacted gall stones.

Stents can also be used to restore biliary continuity after unintended surgical transection of the bile duct, before formal surgical repair.

A strategy for the investigation of the jaundiced patient is given in Figure 4.

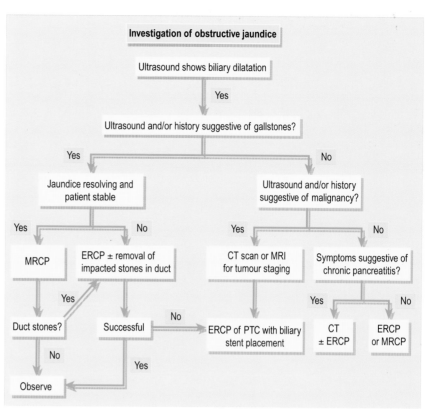

Fig. 4 **Flowchart** of investigation of obstructive jaundice.

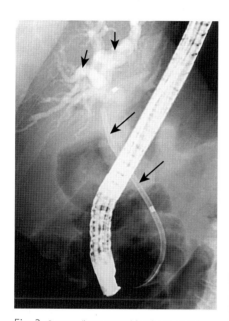

Fig. 3 **A stent** (long arrows) has been paced across a malignant bile duct stricture at endoscopic retrograde cholangiopancreatography. Note the dilated contrast-filled intrahepatic biliary tree (short arrows).

Obstructive jaundice

- Ultrasound is the initial imaging investigation in the jaundiced patient and detects biliary obstruction.
- Endoscopic retrograde cholangiopancreatography (ERCP) allows both diagnosis and therapy in obstructive jaundice.
- Magnetic resonance cholangiopancreatography is a non-invasive alternative to ERCP with almost equal diagnostic ability.
- Computed tomography or magnetic resonance imaging should be performed if an underlying malignancy is suspected.
- Both ERCP and percutaneous transhepatic cholangiography can be used to deploy biliary stents to relieve obstruction, particularly in malignant conditions.

Disorders of the pancreas

The pancreas is a retroperitoneal organ situated in the upper abdomen that has vital exocrine and endocrine functions. Patients with disorders of the pancreas present with a variety of symptoms and signs depending on the underlying pathological process, including pain, malabsorption and diabetes mellitus.

Acute pancreatitis

Gallstones and alcohol underlie most cases of acute pancreatitis, although there are many other precipitants (Box 1).

Pathologically, there is self-perpetuating pancreatic inflammation that is often mild, but may progress to pancreatic haemorrhage and necrosis with widespread intra-abdominal and retroperitoneal fluid collections. In severe cases the mortality may be up to 20%, due to progressive multi-organ failure.

The diagnosis of pancreatitis is usually made clinically based on a history of epigastric pain together with a raised blood amylase. In mild cases, the role of imaging is to exclude a gallstone aetiology and ultrasound is the investigation of choice. The presence of biliary dilatation strongly suggests impacted gallstones within the bile duct. This can be confirmed with either endoscopic retrograde cholangiopancreatography (ERCP) or magnetic resonance cholangiopancreatography (MRCP), the former, although more invasive, having the advantage of allowing removal of impacted stones.

In more severe pancreatitis, a plain abdominal X-ray is frequently performed but is often unhelpful, although it may show a localized ileus with duodenal dilatation in addition to a left-sided pleural effusion.

Imaging aims to assess the complications of pancreatitis, which include intra-abdominal fluid collections and abscesses, pseudoaneurysms, splenic vein thrombosis, and pancreatic necrosis.

Ultrasound may show some of these complications but its sensitivity is limited by overlying bowel gas and a contrast-enhanced computed tomography (CT) scan is the investigation of choice (Fig. 1). Necrotic pancreas does not enhance following injection of intravenous contrast medium on CT and the extent of non-enhancing pancreas gives a good guide to eventual prognosis (Fig. 2). Magnetic resonance imaging (MRI) gives similar information to CT and its use may be preferred in young patients for whom repeated CT scanning carries a significant radiation burden.

Chronic pancreatitis

Chronic pancreatitis is a continuing inflammatory disease of the pancreas characterized by irreversible structural change, typically causing pain and loss of pancreatic function.

Alcohol abuse is by far the commonest aetiology, but developmental abnormalities of the pancreas and tumours should always be borne in mind.

The hallmark of chronic pancreatitis is dilatation and beading of the pancreatic duct, often with associated calcification within the duct and pancreatic parenchyma. The disease may be complicated by formation of well-defined fluid collections (pseudocysts), which may be large enough to cause biliary or gastric outlet obstruction.

The plain abdominal film may show calcification in up to 40% of patients (Fig. 3), but unenhanced CT is the initial investigation of choice (intravenous contrast may mask calcification), with very high sensitivity for pancreatic calcification, duct dilatation and pseudocyst formation (Fig. 4). If CT is normal and clinical suspicion remains high, then ERCP can demonstrate subtle abnormalities of the pancreatic duct to clinch the diagnosis (Fig. 5).

MRCP is a viable alternative to demonstrate an abnormal pancreatic duct. Ultrasound may demonstrate a dilated duct and is useful when

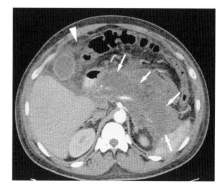

Fig. 2 **Contrast-enhanced computed tomography scan through the pancreas** demonstrates non-enhancement of the gland (arrows) indicating significant necrosis. Note the mesenteric inflammation (arrowhead).

Box 1 Causes of pancreatitis

- Gallstones
- Alcohol
- Drugs (e.g. steroids)
- Hyperlipidaemia
- Viral infection (e.g. mumps)
- Trauma.

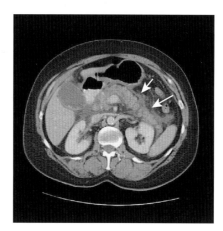

Fig. 1 **Contrast-enhanced computed tomography scan through the upper abdomen** demonstrates mesenteric inflammation and fluid (arrows) immediately adjacent to the body and tail of the pancreas due to acute pancreatitis.

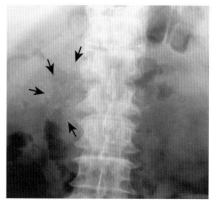

Fig. 3 **Plain abdominal film showing extensive pancreatic calcification** (arrows) due to chronic pancreatitis.

following pseudocyst progression, but is relatively insensitive to the early changes of chronic pancreatitis.

Pancreatic tumours

Adenocarcinoma accounts for over 80% of pancreatic neoplasms, with rarer tumours including mucinous cystic tumours and islet-cell tumours. Patients are usually aged over 60 years and typically present with weight loss and progressive jaundice (because up to 70% of tumours occur in the pancreatic head, through which the common bile duct runs; see pp 60–61).

Ultrasound is often the initial investigation when pancreatic carcinoma is suspected. A low echogenicity mass with dilatation of both common bile and pancreatic ducts ('double duct sign') is typical. However, tumours in the pancreatic body and tail, although often visible (Fig. 6), are less easily seen with ultrasound, because they are obscured by overlying gastric gas.

Contrast-enhanced CT is the investigation of choice in staging patients with a cancer seen on ultrasound or excluding a neoplasm if the ultrasound is equivocal. The CT can give information regarding both vascular invasion and metastatic spread, both of which deem the patient inoperable (Fig. 7).

MRI may be slightly better than CT in staging pancreatic cancer, but is not as widely available. In some patients imaging cannot differentiate between focal pancreatitis and a tumour, and ultrasound- or CT-guided biopsy is required. ERCP and percutaneous transhepatic cholangiography (PTC) mainly have a role in placing biliary stents to relieve jaundice (see pp 60–61).

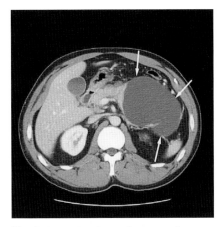

Fig. 4 **Contrast-enhanced computed tomography scan through the pancreas** demonstrates a large well-defined pseudocyst (arrows) due to chronic pancreatitis.

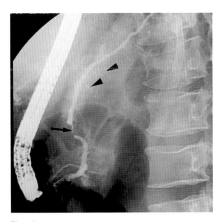

Fig. 5 **Endoscopic retrograde cholangiopancreatography** study demonstrates irregularity and stricturing (arrow) of the main pancreatic duct due to chronic pancreatitis. Note filling of dilated side branches (arrowheads).

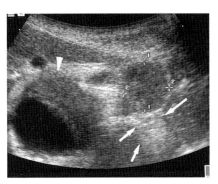

Fig. 6 **Ultrasound of the upper abdomen** demonstrates a well-defined mass (crosses) arising from the pancreas (arrows). Note the incidental aortic aneurysm (arrowhead).

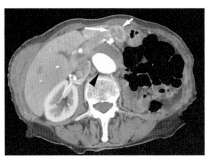

Fig. 7 **Contrast-enhanced CT scan through the pancreas** demonstrates a large heterogeneously enhancing mass (arrows) arising from the body of the gland which proved to be an inoperable primary pancreatic carcinoma.

Disorders of the pancreas

- Mild pancreatitis is a clinical diagnosis and ultrasound is reserved to exclude a gallstone aetiology.

- Computed tomography (CT) is the investigation of choice in severe pancreatitis to look for pancreatic necrosis and associated complications.

- The hallmark of chronic pancreatitis is dilatation and beading of the pancreatic duct, often associated with calcification, and is best seen on endoscopic retrograde cholangiopancreatography (ERCP) or CT.

- Pancreatic cancer commonly presents with weight loss and jaundice, and is best imaged with CT or magnetic resonance imaging (MRI).

Bowel obstruction

There are many causes of bowel obstruction, both of the small and large intestine (Table 1). Patients present with colicky abdominal pain, distension, nausea and vomiting, and constipation.

On examination there may be tinkling bowel sounds in a distended abdomen or, in advanced cases, bowel sounds may be absent altogether. If the obstruction is due to an incarcerated hernia, a tender lump may be palpable at the inguinal or hernial orifices.

Imaging aims to confirm the presence of bowel obstruction, define the level of obstruction, identify the cause, and detect complications such as perforation.

Plain radiography

The first investigation when bowel obstruction is suspected is the supine plain abdominal X-ray, together with an erect chest film if perforation is a possibility. Obstructed bowel appears as dilated gas filled loops with multiple air-fluid levels seen on erect films.

Occasionally, all the dilated bowel may be fluid filled and not visible on a plain X-ray and further imaging with contrast studies, computed tomography (CT) or ultrasound may be needed to demonstrate dilated bowel.

Table 1 **Causes of bowel obstruction**		
Extrinsic	**Bowel wall**	**Intraluminal**
Adhesions	Neoplasia	Intussusception
Hernia	Strictures: inflammatory, radiation, chemical	Foreign body
Volvulus	Intestinal ischaemia	Gallstone ileus
Inflammation/abscess		
Malignant infiltration (e.g. peritoneal deposits)		

The distinction between dilated small bowel and colon is occasionally very difficult. Obstructed small bowel tends to lie centrally in the abdomen, have thin valvulae conniventes (which usually form complete lines across the bowel), and tends to measure 3–5 cm in diameter (Fig. 1).

Colon, however, tends to lie peripherally, has thick haustra (which do not cross the whole bowel lumen), and may measure over 5 cm in diameter. If the ileocecal valve is incompetent, gas from an obstructed colon may reflux into the small bowel, resulting in both dilated large and small bowel. While small bowel obstruction classically leads to a collapsed, empty colon, in the early stages the colon may still contain faecal residue and gas, resulting in diagnostic confusion.

Pneumoperitoneum

The presence of air in the peritoneal cavity is most often due to perforation of an abdominal viscus, and is a very important and serious finding since most patients with a pneumoperitoneum will require emergency surgery.

The most common finding is air under the diaphragms on the erect chest X-ray (Fig. 2). Other signs include a linear or oval collection of air, often under the liver, and visualization of the outer as well as the inner wall of a bowel loop (Rigler's sign). Sometimes, routine X-rays will be normal despite a pneumoperitoneum. If the diagnosis is strongly suspected, a film taken with the patient lying on the left side may demonstrate the free air overlying the liver. Abdominal CT is extremely sensitive for even small volumes of free gas and should be requested when the plain film is normal in the face of high clinical suspicion.

Investigation of bowel obstruction

Some causes of bowel obstruction have specific appearances on plain X-rays and can be confidently diagnosed. For example, in sigmoid volvulus a massively distended U-shaped sigmoid loop is seen pointing towards the left iliac fossa, often overlapping the liver and descending colon (Fig. 3).

Most causes of bowel obstruction cannot be differentiated on plain films, although not all require further investigation.

Many cases of small bowel obstruction are due to adhesions from

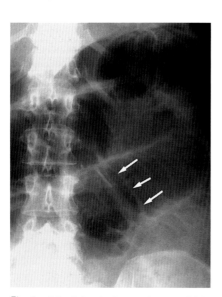

Fig. 1 **Plain abdominal X-ray shows multiple loops of dilated small bowel** due to adhesional obstruction. Note how the valvulae conniventes (arrows) cross the whole width of the dilated bowel.

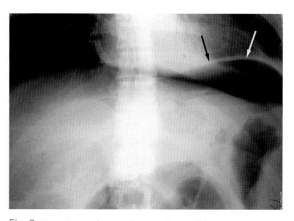

Fig. 2 **Erect X-ray shows a large volume of free intraperitoneal air** outlining the left hemi-diaphragm (arrows).

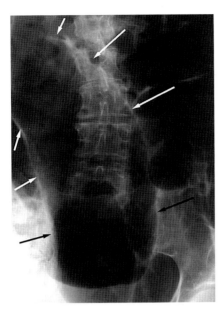

Fig. 3 **Plain abdominal film from a patient with abdominal pain and absolute constipation** shows a massively dilated bowel loop (arrows), pointing to the left iliac fossa. The features are typical of a sigmoid volvulus.

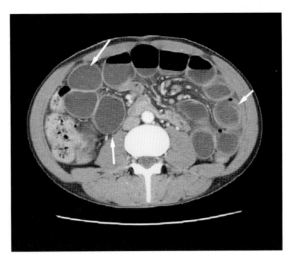

Fig. 4 **Contrast-enhanced computed tomography scan through the abdomen** shows multiple dilated bowel loops (arrows) due to small bowel obstruction.

previous surgery or peritoneal inflammation and are usually managed conservatively without surgical intervention. The next most common cause of obstruction is hernias, which again are nearly always managed surgically without the need for further imaging.

If further diagnostic information is required prior to treatment, then the two most useful investigations are contrast studies and CT scanning. Ultrasound has a more limited role.

If there is doubt as to whether the obstruction is at the level of the small bowel or colon, a contrast enema should be performed to exclude an obstructing lesion in the colon such as a carcinoma, diverticular stricture or volvulus. Barium should not be used as it may become impacted and is dangerous if it enters the peritoneal cavity via an unsuspected perforation or during subsequent surgery.

If the colon is normal or the plain film shows unequivocal small bowel obstruction, an oral contrast study may be performed. This can demonstrate the level of the obstruction and may diagnose the cause. There is some evidence that use of ionic contrast medium may be actually therapeutic by drawing fluid into the bowel and helping the obstruction to resolve.

CT scanning of the abdomen can be very useful in elucidating the level and cause of bowel obstruction (Fig. 4). It can demonstrate tumours, abscesses, diverticular disease, volvulus and hernias. In addition, it is very sensitive for the presence of small amounts of intraperitoneal air and can suggest complications such as bowel

ischaemia. It is, however, a relatively expensive test involving a significant radiation dose and, most importantly, should not delay the passage of a sick patient to the operating theatre. A comparison of the features of various imaging modalities is shown in Table 2.

Table 2 **Comparison of imaging modalities in suspected bowel obstruction**

Feature	Plain film	Contrast study	CT scan
Radiation dose	+	++	+++
Diagnosing obstruction	++	+++	++
Demonstrating cause	+/−	+	+++
Demonstrating perforation	++	+	+++
Demonstrating complications, e.g. ischaemia	−	+	++

Bowel obstruction

■ Supine abdominal and erect chest X-rays are the initial investigations for suspected bowel obstruction.

■ Dilated small bowel tends to lie centrally whereas dilated colon lies peripherally.

■ A pneumoperitoneum is a surgical emergency and most easily diagnosed with an erect chest X-ray.

■ A contrast enema is a simple way of assessing possible colonic obstruction, but barium should not be used if there is a risk of perforation.

■ Computed tomography is reserved for patients not undergoing immediate surgery in whom the diagnosis is unclear.

Tumours and polyps of the colon

Histological types

There are several histological varieties of colonic polyps (Table 1). Radiology, on the whole, cannot distinguish between the types, although some polyps, such as post-inflammatory, have a classical radiological appearance (Fig. 1).

Adenomatous polyps

Because of the risk of malignant transformation to colorectal cancer, colonic adenomas are clinically by far the most important polyps. The risk of developing malignancy is related to the size of the polyp, being 1% in polyps <1 cm, but increasing to 10% in polyps >1 cm.

The conversion into invasive cancer occurs in approximately 2.5 polyps per 1000 per year and takes several years, involving multiple additive genetic mutations. Most adenomas occur in middle age, although patients with familial adenomatous polyposis (FAP), a rare but well-recognized dominantly inherited condition, develop multiple adenomas in adolescence and invariably develop carcinoma unless the colon is removed. Most patients with polyps are asymptomatic, but a few may present with rectal bleeding or a positive faecal occult blood test.

There is strong evidence that removing polyps during endoscopy decreases the risk of subsequently developing colonic carcinoma.

Table 1 Histological varieties of colonic polyps	
Histological type	**Groups**
Neoplastic	Adenomas, carcinoma, lymphoma
Inflammatory	Post-infection or inflammatory bowel disease
Hamartomatous	Peutz-Jegher, juvenile polyposis, Cowdens syndrome
Metaplastic	

Imaging of the colon

Fibre-optic endoscopy remains the gold standard for the detection of colonic polyps and tumours. The technique is, however, highly operator dependent and carries a small risk of colonic perforation with its associated morbidity and mortality.

The standard radiological investigation for imaging the colonic mucosa is the double contrast barium enema. Patients undergo full bowel preparation before the test and barium is introduced into the empty colon.

The double-contrast effect is achieved by distending the barium-coated colon with gas such that the mucosa is seen as a thin white line during fluoroscopy. Any mucosal lesion such as a polyp stands out from the surrounding normal mucosa (Fig. 2).

The sensitivity of the barium enema is limited by the adequacy of bowel preparation and coexisting bowel pathology such as diverticular disease. Patients must be able to tolerate bowel cleansing, be continent, and be relatively mobile, such that elderly or infirm patients may be unsuitable for the test.

In recent years a new method for imaging the colon called computed tomography (CT) colonography has been developed. Patients with a cleansed and gas-distended colon undergo CT scanning and the resulting images can be displayed in 3-D, mimicking the view of the endoscopist (Fig. 3). In the future, it may be possible to perform this technique without cleansing the colon, because computer software can 'subtract' bowel contents from the CT image leaving a clean mucosal surface.

Carcinoma of the colon

Colonic cancer is the second most common malignancy in the Western world. Most tumours are adenocarcinoma and some 60% occur in the rectum or sigmoid. Patients may present with bowel obstruction (see p. 64), weight loss, a change in bowel

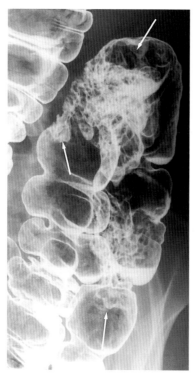

Fig. 1 **View of the descending colon** from a double-contrast barium enema demonstrates multiple filling defects (arrows), the morphology of which is typical of post-inflammatory polyposis.

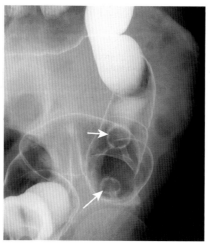

Fig. 2 **Spot view from a double-contrast barium enema** shows two stalked adenomatous polyps (arrows) in the sigmoid colon.

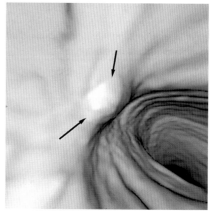

Fig. 3 **Rendered 3-D endoluminal view** from a computed tomography colonography study shows a small polyp (arrows).

habit, rectal bleeding or a palpable abdominal mass.

The barium enema is the most commonly performed radiological investigation for cancer, with sensitivity for detection of over 90%. The classical appearance on the barium enema is an 'apple-core' stricture (Fig. 4) or intraluminal mass, although appearances may be more subtle. Similar appearances are seen with CT colonography.

Contrast-enhanced CT scanning of patients with an unprepared colon is a good alternative in those patients not able to tolerate a barium enema or colonoscopy (Fig. 5).

CT scanning has the advantage of providing some information regarding the stage of the cancer such as the presence of lymphadenopathy or liver metastasis. Ultrasound of the liver is a good imaging alternative in staging patients due to undergo surgical resection of the cancer.

In patients with rectal cancer, accurate pre-operative staging helps plan therapy, particularly pre-operative radiotherapy. Both magnetic resonance imaging (MRI) (Fig. 6) and transrectal ultrasonography allow detection of tumour spread through the bowel wall, although both techniques are

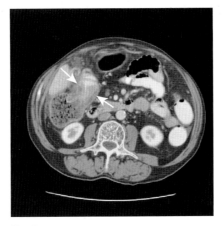

Fig. 5 **Contrast-enhanced computed tomography scan** through the upper abdomen demonstrates a heterogeneously enhancing mass (arrows) at the hepatic flexure proven to be a colonic carcinoma.

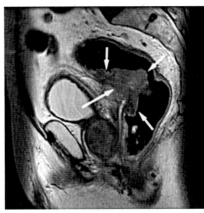

Fig. 6 **Sagittal magnetic resonance sequence** through the pelvis demonstrates a large rectal cancer (arrows).

relatively inaccurate at predicting lymph-node involvement.

Both CT and MRI are useful in investigating patients suspected of having tumour recurrence, although differentiation from postoperative fibrosis may sometimes be difficult. CT-guided biopsy may be required in some cases. Positron emitting tomography (PET) scanning may also have a role by identifying metabolically active tumour.

Colonic stenting

Patients presenting with malignant large bowel obstruction may be too ill to undergo immediate surgery or may have such advanced disease that surgery is inappropriate. The obstruction can be relieved by placing a metallic stent across the stricture, using fluoroscopic guidance. The procedure is frequently a combined procedure between the radiologist and endoscopist.

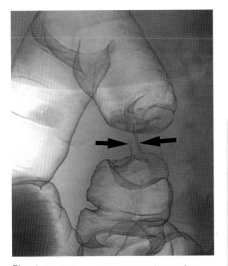

Fig. 4 **Spot view of the descending colon** from a double contrast barium enema shows the typical 'apple-core' appearances of colonic carcinoma (arrows).

Tumours and polyps of the colon

- Adenomatous polyps of the colon are clinically important as they may progress to colonic cancer.
- Colonoscopy remains the gold standard for diagnosis and removal of colonic polyps, although barium enema and computed tomography (CT) colonography are radiological alternatives.
- Colonic cancer typically appears as an 'apple core' stricture or intraluminal mass on barium enema.
- Unprepared CT scan is a good alternative for diagnosing cancer in patients too frail to undergo bowel preparation.
- Magnetic resonance imaging or trans-rectal ultrasound is indicated to locally stage rectal cancer prior to treatment planning.
- Colonic stenting may provide palliation in patients with advanced disease in whom surgery is inappropriate.

Diverticular disease of the colon and appendicitis

Colonic diverticula are acquired out-pouchings of colonic mucosa through the bowel wall, thought to occur secondary to increased intra-colonic pressure. They occur in between the taenia coli at the points of penetration of blood vessels and are associated with a marked increase in elastin within the taenia, giving the affected bowel a shortened concertina-like appearance.

Diverticular disease is rare below age 35 years, but between 30% and 50% of older adults are affected. The disease is associated with the low fibre, highly-refined Western diet and typically affects the left colon, particularly the sigmoid.

In oriental races, however, the diverticula are mainly located in the right colon. While diverticular disease is often asymptomatic, patients may complain of irritable-bowel-like symptoms or present with complications.

Complications of diverticular disease

The most common complications are shown in Box 1.

There is no evidence that diverticular disease predisposes to colonic cancer, but the anatomic distortion caused means that co-existing polyps and cancer can be difficult to diagnose using imaging techniques.

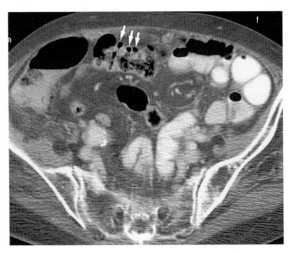

Fig. 2 **Contrast-enhanced computed tomography scan** through the upper pelvis shows gas-filled pockets (arrows) arising from the colon due to diverticula.

Imaging of diverticular disease

Nearly every imaging technique has a role in investigating diverticular disease and the choice of modality depends very much on the clinical presentation.

Patients with longstanding symptoms, such as abdominal pain, rectal bleeding and irregular bowel habit, may have underlying diverticular disease. The radiological modality of choice is the barium enema, where diverticula are seen as small out-pouches from the colonic wall (Fig. 1). Distortion and effacement of the bowel may suggest a complicating abscess. Diverticula are often incidental findings on computed tomography

(CT) scans performed for other reasons (Fig. 2).

In contrast, patients with acute diverticulitis typically present with sudden left-sided abdominal pain and

---

Box 1 Complications of diverticular disease

- Diverticulitis
- Perforation and peritonitis
- Fistula formation – into bladder, vagina or skin
- Bleeding
- Stricture formation and obstruction.

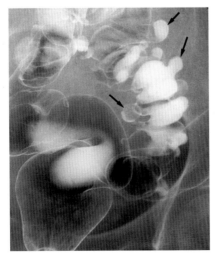

Fig. 1 **Spot view from a double-contrast barium enema** shows multiple outpouchings (arrows) due to diverticula.

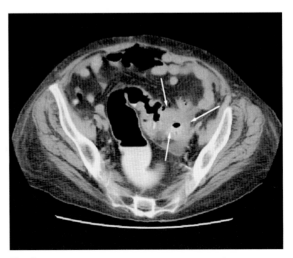

Fig. 3 **Contrast-enhanced computed tomography scan** through the pelvis demonstrates a thick-walled thickened abscess (arrows) due to acute sigmoid diverticulitis.

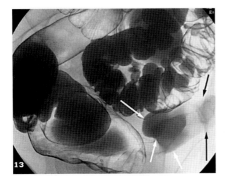

Fig. 4 **Spot view from a double-contrast barium enema** shows contrast medium within the bladder (arrows) due to fistulation from sigmoid diverticular disease.

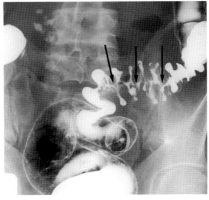

Fig. 5 **Spot view from a double-contrast barium enema** demonstrates a sigmoid stricture (arrows) secondary to diverticular disease.

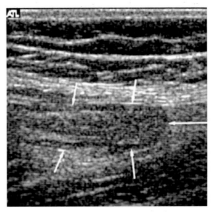

Fig. 6 **Ultrasound of the right iliac fossa** demonstrates a thick-walled distended appendix (arrows) due to acute appendicitis.

fever, and exhibit left-sided abdominal tenderness. The diagnosis is often made clinically and imaging in the acute stage is reserved for those patients who have more severe symptoms or who fail to settle with conservative management. The main role of imaging is to confirm the diagnosis and detect associated abscess formation, which may require percutaneous drainage or surgical evacuation. Ultrasound may detect collections but is highly operator dependent and can miss sizeable abscesses, particularly if they contain gas. For this reason, CT scanning is the preferred modality and can demonstrate thickened inflamed colon and any associated abscess, even when small (Fig. 3). Differentiation of acute diverticulitis from colonic cancer may be difficult on CT, both appearing as a short segment of thickened colon.

Fistula formation
The most common site for fistulation is into the bladder, causing symptoms of pneumaturia. A contrast study of the colon is the first-line investigation for both confirming diverticular disease and demonstrating the fistula (Fig. 4). If this is negative, a cystogram may occasionally show the communication.

Both CT and magnetic resonance imaging (MRI) have a role in demonstrating the proximity of bowel to bladder and may show the fistula itself or a pericolic abscess. The presence of air in the bladder on CT in a non-catheterized patient is highly suggestive of a colo-vesical fistula.

Stricture and obstruction
Diverticular strictures are relatively common and may present acutely with bowel obstruction during an acute flare-up, or more chronically with symptoms of subacute obstruction.

In the more chronic setting the barium enema remains the investigation of choice and will commonly demonstrate a relatively long stricture with intact mucosa (Fig. 5). While the appearances are often highly suggestive of a benign aetiology, endoscopy is often needed to confidently exclude neoplasia. In the acute setting an unprepared water-soluble contrast enema should be performed to outline the stricture.

Bleeding
Most bleeding from diverticular disease is inconsequential and intermittent, but, occasionally, patients may present with a life-threatening bleed. Angiography may be useful in demonstrating the site of bleeding and allow therapy by embolizing the bleeding vessel.

Imaging of the appendix
Ultrasound of the right iliac fossa is useful in patients with pain in whom the diagnosis of appendicitis is clinically in doubt, although a negative scan does not fully exclude the diagnosis. An inflamed appendix is seen as a thick-walled, blind-ending 'sausage' shape, often with surrounding fluid (Fig. 6). Localized CT scanning of the lower abdomen is advocated by some, but carries a heavy radiation burden in a young patient population.

Diverticular disease of the colon and appendicitis

- Diverticular disease has a high incidence in Western cultures and typically affects the left colon.
- Complications include inflammation, perforation, abscess, bleeding and strictures.
- Diverticular disease is easily diagnosed using a barium enema, but computed tomography (CT) is indicated for complications such as abscess formation.
- Differentiating complicated diverticular disease from cancer may be difficult on CT.
- A contrast enema or CT both demonstrate fistulation related to diverticular disease.
- Ultrasound has reasonable sensitivity for diagnosis of appendicitis and avoids the risks of radiation from CT but is highly operator dependent.

Gastrointestinal bleeding

Haematemesis (vomiting blood) and melaena (rectal passage of altered blood, usually black and tar-like) signify bleeding from the upper gastrointestinal tract, whereas the passage of fresh blood per rectum is usually from lower bowel. There are many causes of gastrointestinal bleeding, some of which are listed in Table 1.

Table 1 **Causes of gastrointestinal bleeding**	
Upper gastrointestinal tract	**Lower gastrointestinal tract**
Oesophageal varices	Diverticular disease
Oesophagitis and gastritis	Arteriovenous malformations and angiodysplasia
Mallory–Weiss tear	Meckel's diverticulum
Cancers	Cancers and polyps

Investigation of gastrointestinal bleeding

Acute

Serious or life-threatening haemorrhage can be due to any of the causes in Table 1. In cases of acute upper intestinal bleeding, endoscopy is the investigation of choice both for diagnosis and therapy, e.g. banding of oesophageal varices or injection of bleeding ulcers. Radiology has a rather limited role, but computed tomography (CT) or angiography may be useful in demonstrating more unusual causes such as pseudoaneurysms.

Imaging has a much larger role in investigating bleeding from lower down the gut. Both angiography and nuclear medicine techniques are useful and, in addition to the suspected site of bleeding, the choice of test depends both on local availability and expertise.

Radionuclide scanning

The most commonly used nuclear medicine test is the ^{99m}Tc red cell scan. Patients are injected with a radioactive isotope (^{99m}Tc) that binds to red blood cells. Whole abdomen imaging with a gamma camera can commence immediately and carry on for up to 24 hours. Increased radioactivity is seen corresponding to the site of bleeding and bleeding rates as low as 0.5 ml/min can be detected (Fig. 1).

Angiography

Visceral angiography can be used as a first-line investigation in brisk gastrointestinal bleeding (at least 1 ml/min) or may be used to investigate specific sites of bleeding suggested on prior red cell scan or endoscopy.

With the use of specialized angiographic catheters it is possible to

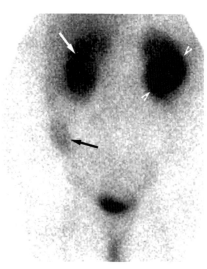

Fig. 1 **^{99m}Tc red cell scan shows abnormal activity in the right iliac fossa** (black arrow) due to bleeding from colonic angiodysplasia. Note normal uptake in the liver (white arrow) and spleen (arrowhead).

selectively inject branches of the main abdominal vessels to precisely define the site of bleeding and allow therapy (Fig. 2).

Various chemicals and coils can be injected into the bleeding vessel to arrest the haemorrhage, avoiding the need for surgery.

Angiodysplasia (abnormal colonic vessels, usually in the right colon) is a common cause of lower gut haemorrhage and while it can be demonstrated on high-quality angiograms, the treatment is usually electrocoagulation during colonoscopy or surgical resection.

Chronic

Chronic gastrointestinal haemorrhage may present as repeated small bleeds, or as iron-deficiency anaemia on blood testing. Upper intestinal endoscopy is more sensitive than the barium meal in demonstrating most causes of blood loss from the stomach and duodenum,

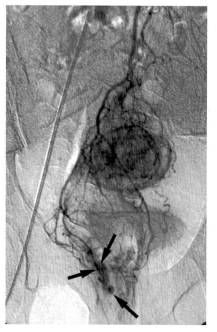

Fig. 2 **Selective angiography of the inferior mesenteric artery** shows active bleeding (arrows) from a haemorrhoidal artery.

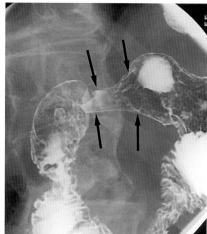

Fig. 3 **Spot view from a double-contrast barium meal** shows irregular stricturing of the gastric antrum due to carcinoma.

and has the advantage of allowing both biopsy and testing for *H. pylori* infection. However, it is invasive and the barium meal is still a good alternative with acceptable sensitivities for detection of advanced peptic ulcer disease and malignancy (Fig. 3).

The barium enema is a very useful alternative to colonoscopy when investigating the colon, with reasonable sensitivities for polyps, cancers and diverticular disease (see pp 66–69). Up to 25% of colonoscopies are incomplete due to technical difficulties, whereas the right colon is imaged in practically all barium enemas. This is important because caecal tumours are a common cause of iron-deficiency anaemia (Fig. 4).

The technique of CT colonography is also very sensitive for detecting causes of colonic blood loss such as diverticular disease and malignancy (Fig. 5), and may replace the barium enema as the standard radiological technique in imaging the colon.

One rare but important cause of recurrent blood loss is a Meckel's diverticulum. This embryological remnant of the vitello-intestinal duct classically occurs 2 feet from the ileocaecal valve and is often

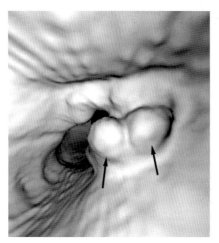

Fig. 5 **Reconstructed CT endoluminal view from CT colonography** shows an irregular, partially obstructing cancer (arrows) in the sigmoid colon.

asymptomatic. However, it may contain ectopic gastric mucosa, which may ulcerate, causing pain and bleeding. The diverticulum may occasionally be seen on barium small bowel follow-through, but the mainstay of diagnosis is via the 'Meckel's scan'. This nuclear medicine test uses intravenously injected ^{99m}Tc

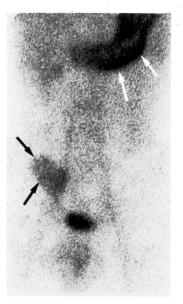

Fig. 6 **^{99m}Tc pertechnetate 'Meckel's' scan** demonstrates simultaneous appearance of activity in the right iliac fossa (black arrows) and stomach (white arrows) due to ectopic gastric mucosa within a Meckel's diverticulum.

pertechnetate, which is taken up by gastric mucosa. A Meckel's diverticulum, therefore, may be revealed by increased activity in the right iliac fossa (Fig. 6).

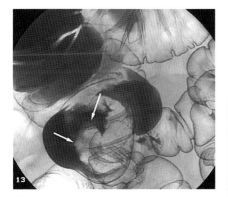

Fig. 4 **Spot view of a double-contrast barium enema** shows a filling defect (arrows) in the caecum due to a large cancer.

Gastrointestinal bleeding

■ Endoscopy remains the investigation of choice for upper gastronintestinal (GI) bleeding.

■ ^{99m}Tc red cell scan is more sensitive but less specific than angiography in diagnosing the cause of ongoing GI bleeding.

■ Angiography allows therapy for GI bleeding with the deployment of coils and glues to occlude bleeding vessels.

■ Barium studies are useful in investigating chronic blood loss.

■ A ^{99m}Tc pertechnetate Meckel's scan is used to detect ectopic gastric mucosa in a Meckel's diverticulum.

Acute abdomen and abdominal trauma

There are numerous causes of the 'acute' abdomen, some of which are listed in Table 1.

Investigating the acute abdomen

In all patients presenting with acute abdominal pain, a thorough history and examination is vital if the correct diagnosis is to be made. Any patient in whom bowel obstruction or perforation is suspected should have a plain abdominal film and an erect chest X-ray to look for dilated loops and free intraperitoneal gas.

In those patients who do not go directly to the operating theatre, the imaging modality of choice thereafter depends on the suspected diagnosis. The investigative pathway for many of the conditions in Table 1 is given in the relevant chapters and those conditions not previously mentioned are discussed below. Suggested first-line imaging investigations for various common causes of acute abdomen are shown in Table 2.

Intestinal ischaemia

Acute small bowel ischaemia is usually caused by sudden occlusion of the superior mesenteric artery by an embolus or thrombosis. Patients are usually elderly and typically present with sudden onset severe abdominal pain and diarrhoea, with the development of a silent non-tender abdomen and shock.

Mortality may be as high as 75% in severe cases and prompt diagnosis and surgical exploration is vital. Imaging often has a role in making the diagnosis because the paucity of physical signs is often out of proportion to the clinical severity of the condition.

The abdominal plain X-ray often shows dilated thick-walled small bowel loops and, in advanced cases, gas may be seen in the bowel wall and portal vein – an ominous sign. Contrast-enhanced computed tomography (CT) is up to 80% sensitive in diagnosing intestinal ischaemia and may demonstrate clot in the superior mesenteric artery, thickened small bowel and possibly gas in the portal venous system. Angiography is

Table 1 Causes of the acute abdomen		
Abdominal organs	**Bowel**	**Other**
Cholecystitis	Bowel obstruction	Intra-abdominal abscess
Pancreatitis	Volvulus	Ruptured aortic aneurysm
Pyelonephritis	Intestinal ischaemia	Ectopic pregnancy
Renal colic	Inflammatory bowel disease	Pelvic inflammatory disease
Liver abscess	Appendicitis	
	Diverticulitis	
	Perforation	

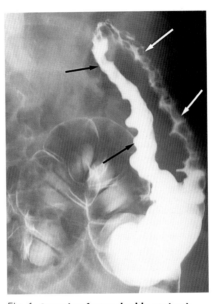

Fig. 1 **Spot view from a double-contrast barium enema** demonstrates a splenic flexure stricture (arrows) secondary to ischaemia.

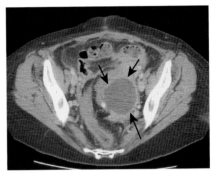

Fig. 2 **Contrast-enhanced computed tomography scan through the pelvis** demonstrates a large abscess due to a perforated sigmoid diverticulum.

invasive but remains the gold standard in equivocal cases.

Colonic ischaemia ('ischaemic colitis') typically occurs at the splenic flexure where there is a watershed between arterial supplies. Bowel wall thickening as a result of submucosal oedema may sometimes be seen on plain films but a contrast enema is more sensitive and elegantly demonstrates the oedematous strictured segment (Fig. 1): 'thumbprinting' is the classical radiological sign.

Intra-abdominal abscess

The most common cause for intra-abdominal abscess formation is recent surgery, often due to an anastamotic leak. Most other abscesses are due to diverticulitis, appendicitis or perforated viscus.

The plain abdominal film may occasionally reveal a gas-containing cavity but has very poor sensitivity overall. Abdominal ultrasound is useful as the initial investigation, particularly for subphrenic collections, and is used to guide percutaneous drainage. However, as a result of gas both within the abscess and in surrounding bowel loops, ultrasound may miss collections particularly in the pelvis, and CT scanning (Fig. 2) or magnetic resonance imaging (MRI) are then indicated.

Table 2 Suggestive first-line imaging tests according to suspected diagnosis		
Condition	**First-line imaging investigation**	**Second-line imaging investigation in complex or equivocal cases**
Bowel obstruction/perforation	Plain films	CT
Cholecystitis	Ultrasound	MRI (e.g. impacted gallstones)
Pancreatitis	CT (in severe cases)	US (to look for gallstones)
Abscess (liver or abdominal)	Ultrasound	CT
Bowel ischaemia	CT	Angiography
Appendicitis	Ultrasound	CT
Diverticulitis	Ultrasound or CT	CT

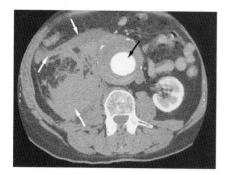

Fig. 3 **Contrast-enhanced computed tomography scan through the abdomen** shows extensive retroperitoneal haematoma (white arrows) due to a leaking aortic aneurysm (black arrow).

Nuclear medicine has a complementary role, with ^{111}In-labelled white-cell scanning having good sensitivity for the detection of intra-abdominal sepsis, particularly if other tests are equivocal.

Leaking aortic aneurysm

The presence of a palpable pulsatile mass in a shocked patient is highly suggestive of a leaking aortic aneurysm and should prompt laparotomy. However, occasionally imaging may be indicated in a stable patient in whom the diagnosis is in doubt. Ultrasound has excellent sensitivity for demonstrating an aneurysm and this may be enough to prompt surgical exploration when present. Ultrasound is, however, very poor at demonstrating an active leak from an aneurysm and contrast-enhanced CT has much better sensitivity (Fig. 3). The mortality from a leaking aneurysm is very high and surgery should not be delayed for investigations if this will compromise the outcome.

Abdominal trauma

All patients with significant trauma will have plain X-rays of the neck, chest and pelvis. Thereafter, imaging is guided by the extent of suspected injury. Patients who are haemodynamically unstable after blunt abdominal trauma require immediate laparotomy. However, in stable patients suspected of intra-abdominal injury, imaging has a diagnostic role. The plain film is rarely helpful and can often be omitted.

The role of ultrasound is controversial. It has excellent sensitivity for the demonstration of free intraperitoneal fluid, which is useful as a marker of abdominal injury, particularly in the unstable patient, and often prompts surgical exploration or further tests. However, sensitivity for detection of solid-organ injury is only moderate and it is notably insensitive for free intraperitoneal gas and retroperitoneal injury.

The imaging investigation of choice in the stable patient with suspected significant intra-abdominal injury is, therefore, contrast-enhanced CT.

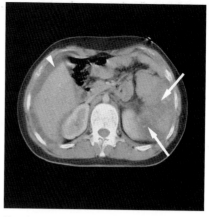

Fig. 4 **Contrast-enhanced computed tomography scan through the upper abdomen** in a patient after major trauma. Laceration of the spleen is well seen (arrows). Note the fluid around the liver (arrowhead) due to free intraperitoneal blood.

Injuries to solid organs such as the liver, kidneys and spleen are well shown (Fig. 4), as is free air, and associated fractures of the spine and pelvis can also be assessed. Many injuries can be managed conservatively in the stable patient and so CT often spares the patient exploratory surgery.

Acute abdomen and abdominal trauma

- Correct diagnosis of acute abdominal pain requires careful history and examination with the judicious use of radiological investigations.
- Patients with intestinal ischaemia often have few physical signs despite the severity of the condition and computed tomography (CT) may aid diagnosis.
- Intra-abdominal abscesses may be seen with ultrasound but CT is more sensitive and specific.
- Imaging should not delay laparotomy in cases of suspected leaking aortic aneurysm, but both ultrasound and CT may aid diagnosis where appropriate.
- In cases of abdominal trauma, ultrasound has excellent sensitivity in demonstrating intraperitoneal blood, but CT has overall better diagnostic accuracy.

Inflammatory bowel disease

Crohn's disease

Crohn's disease is a chronic granulomatous inflammatory disorder of unknown aetiology that can affect any part of the alimentary tract from the mouth to the anus. The disease mainly affects young adults, although it may present for the first time in older individuals. Patients typically present with pain, diarrhoea and weight loss.

Inflammation frequently affects the whole bowel wall (i.e. 'transmural', unlike ulcerative colitis) and leads to the formation of deep ulceration, often with so-called 'cobblestoning' of the mucosa, fistulation and stricture formation. The terminal ileum is particularly affected (approximately 50%) and perianal fistulae and abscesses are also common. The colon is affected in approximately 25% of patients.

Perhaps the most characteristic feature of Crohn's disease is the non-continuous involvement of the bowel with so-called skip lesions between normal intervening segments.

Ulcerative colitis

Ulcerative colitis is an idiopathic recurrent inflammatory disease of the large bowel, always involving the rectum. The rest of the alimentary tract is not directly involved. The inflammatory process does not involve the full thickness of the bowel wall and so fistulation is rare. Patients present with blood and mucus per rectum, often with diarrhoea and fever.

A comparison between Crohn's disease and ulcerative colitis is shown in Table 1, and there may be considerable difficulty distinguishing between the two in some cases.

Imaging in inflammatory bowel disease

Although the diagnosis of inflammatory bowel disease is ultimately made with biopsy and histology, imaging has a major role.

Plain radiography

In patients with colitis the plain film may show lack of faecal residue within

Table 1 Comparison between Crohn's disease and ulcerative colitis		
Pathology	**Ulcerative colitis**	**Crohn's disease**
Distribution	Continuous	Skip lesions
Rectal involvement	Always	About 20%
Depth of wall involved	Mainly mucosal	Transmural
Granuloma	Absent	Characteristic
Complications		
Strictures	Unusual: mainly longstanding disease	Common and often multiple
Fistulae	Very rare	Common
Anal/perianal lesions	Uncommon	Common
Toxic megacolon	Relatively common	Unusual
Malignant transformation	High risk	Lower risk

the colon in combination with a thickened bowel wall. *Toxic dilatation* of the colon occurs in a small number of patients with inflammatory bowel disease (predominately ulcerative colitis) who are acutely ill and it is very important to recognize it since colonic perforation is common. The colon is gas filled and distended with haustral blunting and mucosal thickening (Fig. 1). The patient is at an especially high risk of perforation when the transverse colon diameter exceeds 5.5 cm, a finding that indicates emergency colectomy may be necessary.

Contrast studies

Although the plain film may show thickened dilated loops in Crohn's disease, the mainstay for diagnosis and assessment of disease extent in the small bowel is the barium follow-through. Patients drink barium (approximately 600 ml) and then the small bowel is examined by compressing the abdomen during X-ray fluoroscopy. Ulceration (Fig. 2), fold thickening, stricture formation (Fig. 3), and fistulation can all be seen with a good-quality study.

The colon can be examined by double-contrast barium enema, which elegantly demonstrates ulceration and stricturing. Inflammatory bowel disease, particularly longstanding ulcerative colitis, is associated with an increased risk of colonic malignancy (see p. 66). Patients with Crohn's disease additionally have a risk of small bowel malignancy.

In patients with severe colitis in whom the colon is often empty due to diarrhoea, there may be no need to give bowel preparation before radiological contrast: the instant enema. In patients at risk of perforation or in whom biopsy has recently been performed, barium should *not* be used because it causes severe peritoneal inflammation and

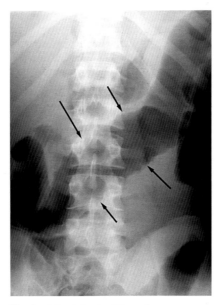

Fig. 1 **Plain abdominal X-ray demonstrates toxic megacolon** (arrows) due to fulminant colitis.

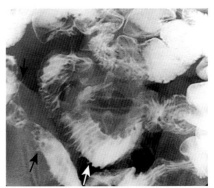

Fig. 2 **Compression spot view from a barium follow-through** shows deep small bowel ulceration (arrows) due to Crohn's disease.

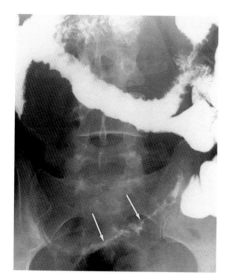

Fig. 3 **X-ray from a barium follow-through** demonstrates a long small-bowel stricture (arrows) due to Crohn's disease.

those with suspected intra-abdominal collections, which may require either surgical or percutaneous drainage (Fig. 5). CT also has a role in imaging those patients with fistulae, particularly into another abdominal viscus such as the bladder. Associated lymphadenopathy and mesenteric fat hypertrophy is often seen on CT.

Magnetic resonance imaging

Like CT, magnetic resonance imaging (MRI) demonstrates the bowel wall thickening in patients with inflammatory bowel disease and has a role in detection of fistulae and collections, particularly in young patients where the radiation dose of a CT scan must be taken into consideration.

A major role for MRI is to image perianal sepsis and fistulae common in Crohn's disease. MRI can reveal fistulae and abscesses that are unsuspected on clinical examination and is able to document the full extent of sepsis prior to surgical treatment (Fig. 6)

Nuclear medicine

Once the diagnosis of inflammatory bowel disease has been established, 99mTc or ^{111}In-labelled white-cell scanning may be very useful for assessing the extent and activity of the disease, particularly in response to treatment. After injection, patients are scanned at intervals of 1 and 4 hours, with diseased bowel showing increased wall uptake.

fibrosis if it escapes from the bowel lumen: water-soluble contrast should be used instead.

Ultrasound

Wall thickening (Fig. 4), mesenteric inflammation, intra-abdominal collections, and even fistulation can be seen using ultrasound.

Computed tomography

Although contrast-enhanced computed tomography (CT) can demonstrate bowel wall thickening in patients with inflammatory bowel disease, it is mainly reserved for the investigation of

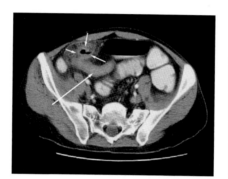

Fig. 5 **Contrast-enhanced computed tomography scan through the pelvis** shows thickened terminal ileum (long arrow) due to Crohn's disease with a small complicating abscess (short arrows).

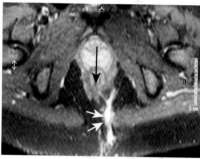

Fig. 6 **Axial magnetic resonance sequence through the perineum** demonstrates a fistula (short arrows) arising from the anal canal (long arrow).

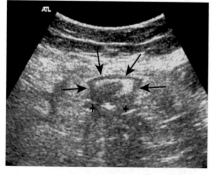

Fig. 4 **Ultrasound of the right iliac fossa** demonstrates thick-walled terminal ileum in cross-section (arrows) due to Crohn's disease with a small abscess (crosses).

Inflammatory bowel disease

- Crohn's disease is a transmural non-contiguous inflammatory condition of the alimentary tract.

- Ulcerative colitis is a contiguous superficial inflammatory condition of the colon, always involving the rectum.

- Toxic megacolon has an associated high risk of perforation and is best assessed with a plain abdominal X-ray.

- Barium studies form the mainstay of radiological assessment of inflammatory bowel disease, although computed tomography and magnetic resonance imaging (MRI) give better information regarding extraluminal complications.

- MRI is superior to clinical examination in the assessment of perianal fistulae complicating Crohn's disease.

Intra-abdominal tumours and lymphoma

Previous chapters have dealt with tumours of the abdominal organs such as pancreas, liver and colon. This chapter will deal with those tumours arising within the abdomen that do not arise directly from the solid organs.

Metastasis

The most common form of intra-abdominal malignancy is metastatic spread from a primary tumour either within (e.g. stomach, pancreas or colon) or outside the abdominal cavity (particularly lung, breast and melanoma).

Tumour deposits can occur within the mesentery and omentum (often giving rise to malignant ascites), along the serosal surface of the bowel (which may lead to bowel obstruction) and within abdominal organs, particularly the liver and adrenal glands.

While ultrasound is very useful for examining solid organs and for detecting ascites, it is relatively poor at detecting peritoneal disease. Contrast-enhanced computed tomography (CT) and magnetic resonance imaging (MRI) are both sensitive for demonstrating solid mesenteric deposits (Figs 1 & 2) and are useful in assessing response to treatment.

Stromal tumours

The abdomen contains tissue derived from all three embryonic lineages (ectoderm, mesoderm and endoderm) and as such many varieties of stromal tumours may arise within the abdominal cavity.

Most of these tumours are sarcomatous (e.g. leiomyosarcoma and rhabdomyosarcoma) and most appear as a non-specific soft-tissue mass on CT or MRI. However, liposarcoma has specific features on CT and MRI that allow the diagnosis to be made without the need for biopsy. As the name suggests, the tumours contain fat, which is easily identifiable on both imaging modalities (Fig. 3). Again, both CT and MRI are useful in detecting tumour recurrence after resection.

Desmoid tumours

These unusual tumours are strongly associated with familial adenomatous polyposis (see p. 66) and may be precipitated by abdominal surgery (often the prophylactic colectomy). Although they are benign mesenchymal tumours arising from the small-bowel mesentery, they are locally aggressive and surround and compress neighbouring structures, most commonly small bowel and mesenteric vessels. This can lead to intractable bowel obstruction and inability to resect these tumours because their proximity to vital structures means that they are frequently fatal. Ultrasound can demonstrate desmoids but views may be obscured by bowel gas. Both CT and MRI document the full extent of local spread of the tumour and because patients are often young, MRI is generally preferred to avoid excessive radiation from repeated CT scans (Fig. 4).

Lymphoma

Intra-abdominal lymphoma is most commonly part of a systemic disease process but may occur as a primary tumour of the gastrointestinal tract. Most lymphomas within the abdomen are non-Hodgkin's in type.

Primary lymphoma of the gastrointestinal tract most commonly affects the stomach (Fig. 5), but may also affect the small bowel and colon. The appearance on barium studies (barium meal, follow-through or enema) is variable, as the tumours may be polypoidal, ulcerating or infiltrating, leading to strictures (Fig. 6).

If lymphoma is suspected on a barium study then cross-sectional imaging, usually CT, is indicated that often not only demonstrates the abnormally thickened bowel, but also assesses the degree of spread to local lymph nodes. Such local staging dictates whether the initial treatment is with surgery or chemotherapy.

When the lymphoma is part of a systemic disease, imaging has a vital role in staging in order to guide therapy and monitor treatment. Intra-abdominal lymphoma is often present in the liver and particularly the spleen,

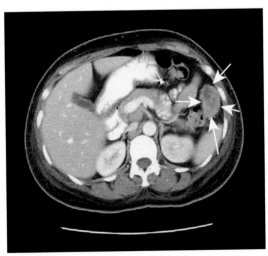

Fig. 1 **Contrast-enhanced computed tomography through the upper abdomen** demonstrates an enhancing mesenteric mass (arrows) due to metastatic ovarian carcinoma.

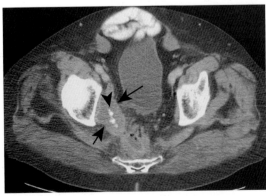

Fig. 2 **Contrast-enhanced computed tomography through the pelvis** shows a mass (arrows) abutting the pelvic side wall containing central calcification (arrowhead). Biopsy proves the lesion to be recurrent rectal cancer.

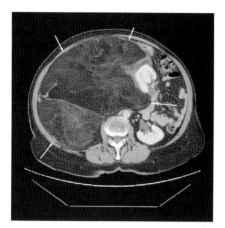

Fig. 3 **Contrast-enhanced computed tomography through the abdomen** shows a large fatty mass (arrows) typical of a liposarcoma.

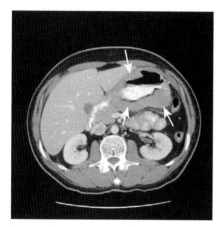

Fig. 5 **Contrast-enhanced computed tomography through the upper abdomen** shows a markedly thick-walled stomach (arrows) due to gastric lymphoma.

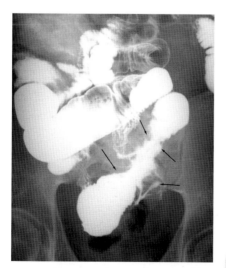

Fig. 6 **Spot film from a small bowel follow-through** demonstrates irregular distorted small bowel (arrows) due to lymphoma. Note the extra-luminal contrast due to cavity formation.

which often appear uniformly enlarged on both ultrasound and CT. The major role of imaging is detecting the involvement of lymph node groups within the abdomen and pelvis.

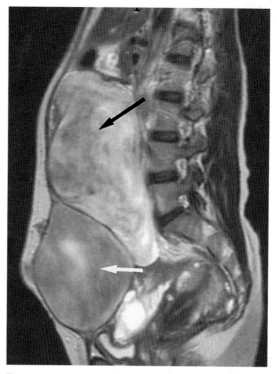

Fig. 4 **Sagittal magnetic resonance imaging sequence through the pelvis** of a patient with familial adenomatous polyposis shows a large desmoid tumour (black arrow) lying above the bladder (white arrow).

Secondary spread to other abdominal organs is less common but does occur and is also well shown with cross-sectional techniques.

While ultrasound gives reliable information regarding solid organs, views of the pelvic sidewall and retroperitoneum are often limited due to bowel gas, decreasing the sensitivity for lymph-node involvement. In this context, CT scanning is again the imaging modality of choice. MRI has a smaller role, as it is generally less available. Both CT and ultrasound can be used to guide diagnostic percutaneous biopsy when this is necessary.

In recent years, positron emission tomography (PET) has found an increasing role in the imaging of malignancy, particularly lymphoma. A glucose analogue labelled with a positron-emitting isotope, typically [18]2-fluoro-2-deoxyglucose, is injected into the patient and accumulates in glucose-avid processes, notably tumours and inflammation. Imaging is then performed in a specialized PET scanner. Studies have shown PET to be more sensitive than either CT or MRI in detecting small volumes of viable tumour and thus aids treatment planning.

Acknowledgements

Thanks are due to Professor C. I. Bartram and Dr V. Goh for supplying many of the images used in this section.

Intra-abdominal tumours and lymphoma

- Most intra-abdominal malignancy is due to metastatic disease and is best diagnosed with computed tomography (CT).

- Stromal tumours are rare and on the whole have non-specific imaging appearances, although liposarcoma has characteristic features on CT and magnetic resonance imaging (MRI).

- Desmoid tumours are associated with familial adenomatous polyposis and are locally aggressive. CT and MRI are the investigations of choice.

- Primary lymphoma of the gastrointestinal tract has a varied appearance on barium studies and CT is often indicated to assess extraluminal spread.

- Most abdominal lymphoma occurs as part of a systemic disease and CT has a pivotal role in staging and monitoring treatment.

Genitourinary System

Imaging techniques used in the investigation of renal disease 1

In practice, patients present with a list of symptoms and, in order to narrow the differential diagnosis, the clinician and the radiologist have to plan a pathway of investigations that will lead most cost-effectively and *care-effectively* to the diagnosis (see Table 1).

Plain radiography

The abdominal plain X-ray (known as the KUB – kidneys, ureters, bladder) includes the renal areas, and must also show the symphysis pubis for calcification in the posterior urethra.

The plain film is used to show calculi, which may be the cause of pain, obstruction, haematuria or infection (Fig. 1).

Spinal disease is also demonstrated on the plain film (Fig. 2). Spina bifida may result in a neuropathic bladder. Metastatic disease from prostate or kidney may also be apparent. In addition, the renal outlines are fairly well demonstrated on the plain film itself, as is the outline of the bladder.

Ultrasound of kidneys and pelvis

Ultrasound (US) is used to assess renal size. The kidneys may be shrunken with chronic renal failure (Fig. 3). Obstructive disease may result in dilatation of the collecting system, again easily visualized with US (Fig. 4).

Tumoral masses are demonstrated and their nature may be assessed using this technique. Benign cysts contain fluid that produces no impedance to US and are thus free of

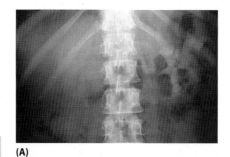

(A)

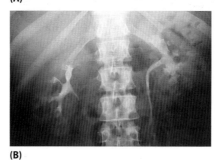

(B)

Fig. 1 **(A) Abdominal plain X-ray (KUB).** A staghorn calculus fills the left pelvicalyceal system. (B) Following injection with contrast medium, the stone is completely hidden by the contrast.

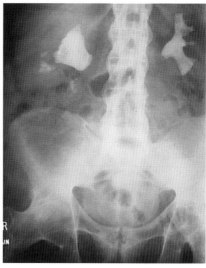

Fig. 2 **Abdominal plain X-ray (KUB).** Large bilateral staghorn calculi: the patient also has ankylosing spondylitis (fused spine, sacro-iliac joints and hips).

Table 1 **Radiological assessment of common pathological processes involving the urinary tract**	
Pathology	Imaging technique
Congenital	
Obstruction	Ultrasound
Trauma	
Avulsed kidney	Computed tomography
Infection	
Tuberculosis	Intravenous urography
Tumour	
Benign – cysts	Ultrasound/computed tomography
Malignant	Computed tomography/magnetic resonance imaging
Metabolic	
Calculi	Intravenous urography/computed tomography

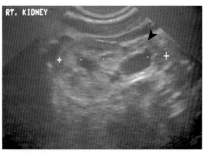

Fig. 3 **Ultrasound showing a small shrunken kidney** with very thin parenchyma over the lower pole (arrowhead).

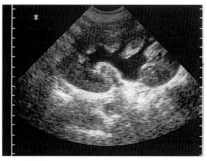

Fig. 4 **Ultrasound demonstrating an echo-free dilated pelvicalyceal system** due to obstruction.

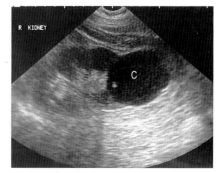

Fig. 5 **Ultrasound of simple anechoic renal cyst** (C) in the lower pole of the right kidney.

internal echoes (Fig. 5). Tumours produce mixed internal echoes.

Computed tomography

This technique also involves injection of intravenous iodinated contrast medium. Axial images are obtained, but reconstructions are available in any plane (Fig. 6). These images are excellent for showing anatomical detail and are especially useful in showing tumours of the urinary tract, as well as other retroperitoneal lesions affecting the kidneys, perhaps causing obstructions. Unfortunately, there is a high dose of ionizing radiation to the patient which, in itself, can have a harmful effect.

Magnetic resonance imaging

This enables the production of cross-sectional anatomy with reconstructions without the use of ionizing radiation. The anatomical detail is perhaps not quite as good as computed tomography (CT) and the technique is rather expensive.

Magnetic resonance angiography

This is a developing technique to show the blood supply to and from the kidneys in place of catheter angiography. The anatomy of the renal vessels is well displayed by this technique.

Catheter angiography

This technique used to be the main method to demonstrate renal vascular abnormalities (Fig. 7), but is now being replaced by CT angiography and magnetic resonance angiography. It involves introducing a fine catheter into a femoral artery and advancing it to the renal artery. By selectively injecting contrast medium, fine anatomical detail of the renal arterial bed can be shown. The method is still the basis for catheter manipulations such as embolization of a traumatic bleed (interventional radiology).

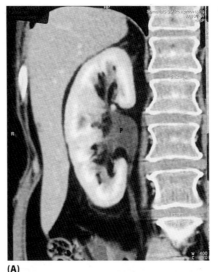

(A)

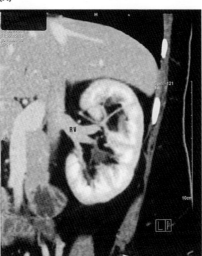

(B)

Fig. 6 **Computed tomography (CT).** (A) CT reconstruction of the right kidney in the coronal plane to show the enhancement of the renal parenchyma immediately after injection of intravenous contrast medium. There is contrast enhancement of the medulla surrounding the papillae; the contrast medium is not yet in the non-opacified pelvis (P). (B) A rotated left posterior view of the right kidney showing the renal vein (RV).

Magnetic resonance urography

This is a urogram using coronal images from magnetic resonance imaging (MRI) and is thus without irradiation, but it is a very expensive technique (Fig. 8).

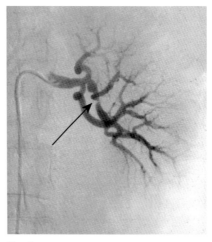

Fig. 7 **Left renal angiogram** showing focal stenosis of lower pole branch (arrow).

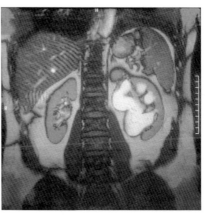

Fig. 8 **Magnetic resonance urogram** showing dilated left collecting system due to obstruction at the pelvi-ureteric junction.

Investigation of renal disease 1

- Abdominal plain X-ray (KUB)
- Ultrasound (US)
- Intravenous urography (IVU)
- Computed tomography (CT)
- Magnetic resonance imaging (MRI)
- Radioisotope imaging.

Imaging techniques used in the investigation of renal disease 2: interventional radiology

Intravenous urography

This technique utilizes intravenous iodinated contrast medium, which is selectively excreted by the kidneys. The renal parenchyma is initially opacified 1–2 mins after injection, followed, at 5–10 mins, by opacification of the renal pelvis, ureters and bladder. The anatomical detail of the renal tract is, therefore, shown. The technique is particularly sensitive at depicting fine abnormalities of the renal calyceal system (Fig. 1A).

Tomography during intravenous urography

By a synchronized movement of the X-ray tube and film during a radiographic exposure, different depths in the body can be focused, thus blurring out unwanted detail of overlying bowel gas or underlying bone (Fig. 1B).

Poor distension of the collecting system can be improved by higher intravenous doses of contrast medium and by applying abdominal compression at 5 mins to squeeze the ureters at the inlet to the pelvis (Fig. 2).

Congenital anomalies can be demonstrated (Fig. 3). Renal masses that may be benign cysts or tumours may be detected, distorting the renal outline and the collecting systems. Obstruction can also be assessed (Fig. 4).

Good renal function is necessary to employ intravenous urography. *Renal failure is often a contraindication to this examination.*

Radionuclide scanning

Various techniques are available that show both anatomy and function. Functional assessment may be total and differential between the two kidneys. Various isotopes are used.

DTPA scan

This uses a filtered isotope and is, therefore, good at assessing pelvicalyceal obstruction. When a diuretic is given, the isotope is not washed out of the obstructed kidney (Fig. 5).

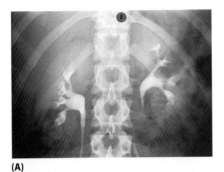
(A)

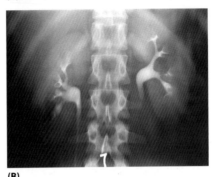
(B)

Fig. 1 **Intravenous urography.** (A) 10-minute post-intravenous contrast medium injection; normal anatomy of collecting systems.
(B) Tomography clears away the overlying bowel gas and gives even better definition.

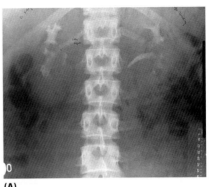
(A)

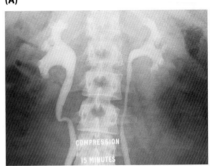
(B)

Fig. 2 **Intravenous urography.** (A) Poor IVU with insufficient contrast medium; thought to have filling defects in the right kidney.
(B) Following high dose of contrast medium and abdominal compression – shows normal anatomy.

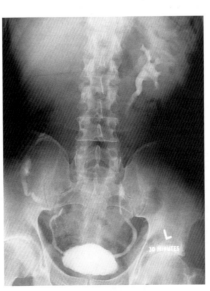

Fig. 3 **Intravenous urography.** A 30-minute film demonstrating a congenital malrotated right pelvic kidney (an incidental finding).

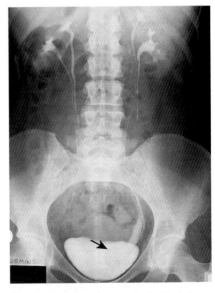

Fig. 4 **Intravenous urography (IVU).** Full length IVU film at 30 mins with bilateral congenital duplication of the collecting systems and ureters. There is a non obstructing ureterocoele on the left (dilated intra-mural portion to the left ureter at the ureteric orifice) (arrow).

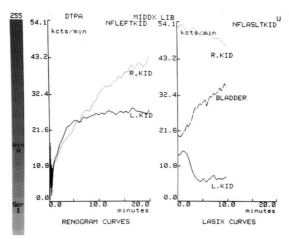

Fig. 5 **DTPA with obstruction to right kidney** – the isotope is not washed out by Lasix.

DMSA scan

This utilizes tubular function and, therefore, is used to assess renal function (Fig. 6).

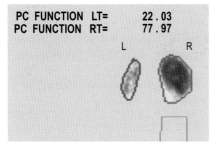

Fig. 6 **DMSA–posterior view.** The right kidney shows 78% function, but the left only 22%.

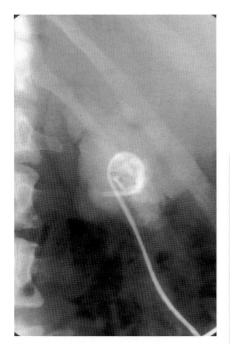

Fig. 7 **Percutaneous nephrostomy** decompressing an obstructed pyonephrosis. A pigtail catheter is coiled in the renal pelvis partly outlined by contrast medium.

MAG3 scan

This assesses tubular function as well as obstruction (see Fig. 2, p. 84).

Interventional radiology

Needle nephrostomy

This is one of the most rewarding aspects of interventional radiology. A patient with a solitary kidney, for example, who drops a stone down a ureter and develops acute failure, pain and a pyonephrosis, requires an immediate decompression to relieve the pain. This will hopefully allow for a full recovery of function and prevent the infected urine leading to a life-threatening Gram-negative septicaemia.

Ultrasound and X-ray guidance allow a needle to be advanced under local anaesthetic into the dilated calyx. Using an angiographic technique, a guide wire is passed through the needle and a pigtail catheter with multiple side holes is advanced over

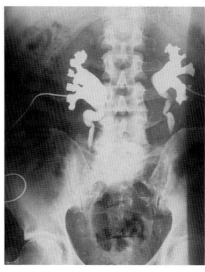

Fig. 8 **Bilateral needle nephrostomies** with bilateral ureteric obstruction due to retroperitoneal fibrosis.

the wire, advanced into the renal pelvis (Fig. 7) and sutured to the skin to allow free external drainage. A urine sample is taken for bacteriology and antibiotic cover given.

Once the kidney is free to drain this way, function usually rapidly returns to normal, unless there has been longstanding obstruction or there is associated infection. When symptoms are stable (1 or 2 days), a contrast nephrostogram can then be performed to identify the level and possible cause of the obstruction (Fig. 8).

Needle nephrostomies are also performed for malignant obstruction prior to surgery or oncology. They are often used for antegrade ureteric stent placement also; this allows internal drainage past an obstruction, which is clearly preferable to long-term nephrostomies.

Investigation of renal disease 2: interventional radiology

Intravenous urography
- The plain film, prior to the examination, shows opaque calculi and also spinal abnormality.
- Intravenous urography is cheap and widely available.
- Abnormalities of the renal outline, pelvicalyceal systems and ureters are shown.
- Sites of obstruction can be identified.
- The bladder and prostatic outlines are easily identified.
- The after-micturition film gives a good indication of bladder function and outlet obstruction.

Ultrasound
- No irradiation.
- Inexpensive.
- Painless.
- Differentiates cyst from tumour.
- First line to check for obstruction.

Renal failure

Patients with renal failure present in two very different ways. Renal failure may be acute or chronic. The diagnosis and management of each is quite different.

Acute or chronic renal failure?

Although the renal failure may be acute, it may actually be superimposed on a more chronic process. Patient examination and electrolyte analysis will diagnose renal insufficiency, but the question to be determined at imaging is whether the kidneys are of normal size (indicating acute renal failure), or small and shrunken (indicating acute renal failure superimposed on the chronic form). In acute failure all treatment must be directed to support those patients who may well recover normal function.

Imaging strategies should concentrate on answering two questions:

1. What is the size of the kidney?
2. Is there an obstruction?

Acute renal failure (Box 1)
This may be:

- *pre-renal*, owing to a drop in blood flow or perfusion to the kidneys, for example, following haemorrhage

Box 1 Causes of acute renal failure

Decreased blood flow
- Trauma
- Surgery
- Septic shock
- Haemorrhage
- Burns
- Dehydration.

Acute tubular necrosis (ATN)
- Acute arterial occlusion of the kidney
- Renal artery stenosis.

Myoglobinuria
- Rhabdomyolysis
- Alcohol abuse
- Crush injury
- Seizures.

Direct injury to the kidney

Urinary-tract obstruction
- Tumours
- Kidney stones.

Disorders of the blood
- Idiopathic thrombocytopenic purpura (ITP)
- Transfusion reaction
- Other haemolytic disorders
- Malignant hypertension
- Bleeding placenta abruptio
- Placenta praevia.

Autoimmune disorders
- Scleroderma.

Haemolytic uraemic syndrome

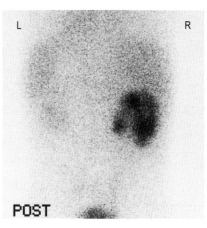

Fig. 2 **A patient with bilateral calculi and long-standing obstruction and infection** – MAG3 radioisotope scan, posterior view. The right kidney is shown with a dilated renal pelvis but there is no function in the left kidney.

- owing to *intrinsic renal failure*, for example, acute tubular dysfunction
- *post-renal*, owing to obstruction, for example, a stone obstructing a solitary kidney.

The immediate challenge to the clinician is to diagnose and treat any pre-renal cause, whereas the immediate challenge to the radiologist is to diagnose or exclude obstruction.

Before the advent of dialysis, a patient presenting with acute intrinsic renal failure had a life expectancy of only 1 week or 2 irrespective of the underlying cause. However, now acute dialysis is available, there is a further diagnostic question. Is the renal dysfunction reversible or irreversible?

Radiological investigations

Plain radiography
An X-ray of the abdomen to include the kidneys, ureters and bladder (KUB) is obtained to exclude calculi.

Ultrasound
This will give an easy, immediate and accurate answer to the questions of size and obstruction in the majority of cases (Fig. 1). In very obese patients it can be difficult to image deep kidneys. Ultrasound will usually detect renal stones, but the ureters are often not seen well at sonography because of the overlying bowel gas.

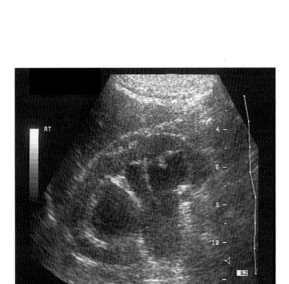

Fig. 1 **Ultrasound of an obtruded kidney** with marked dilatation of the collecting system and some thinning of the parenchyma, i.e. this is not acute. Compare with Fig. 4, p. 80.

Radionuclide scanning
Nuclear medicine gives the best assessment of renal function and is vital in the management of all renal patients. Differential function at isotope scanning shows how each kidney is functioning. Base-line and follow-up of function is well assessed by isotope scanning (Fig. 2).

Computed tomography
This is rarely needed in the acute situation.

Emergency needle nephrostomy

In acute renal failure an emergency needle nephrostomy may be carried out if the following signs are present:

- ultrasound has shown dilated collecting systems (but this may be minimal if acute)
- high serum K^+ – cardiac morbidity
- rising creatinine
- pyrexia and a raised white blood cell count.

A nephrostomy can be delayed if dialysis is at hand, **except** when there is infection – pyonephrosis.

Chronic renal failure (Box 2)
The diagnosis here is usually due to an intrinsic cause such as end-stage failure following reflux nephropathy.

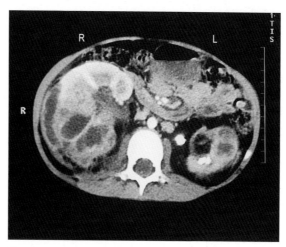

Fig. 3 **A computed tomography scan of the same patient as Fig. 2 following injection of contrast medium** shows the right kidney to have very poor function. Only the anterior parenchyma is perfused (enhanced). Hydronephrosis of the right kidney is shown, whereas the left kidney is shrunken with stones in the calyces blocking the pelvi-ureteric junction.

Even in chronic failure, however, if an obstructive element can be detected, it is worth reversing this to prevent any further deterioration in function.

Radiological investigations

Ultrasound
This is used to assess renal size, parenchymal depth and obstruction (Fig. 1).

Computed tomography
This is extremely useful in giving accurate cross-sectional anatomy of the retroperitoneum to detect any extrinsic cause of chronic obstruction, such as retroperitoneal fibrosis or tumour (Fig. 3).

Radionuclide scanning
This is vital in the follow-up of all cases of renal insufficiency to assess changes in renal function and prognosis during treatment.

Box 2 Causes of chronic renal failure

- Diabetes
- Hypertension
- Glomerulonephritis
- Pyelonephritis
- Polycystic kidney disease
- Alport syndrome
- Reflux nephropathy
- Obstructive neuropathy
- Kidney stones and infection
- Analgesic nephropathy
- Amyloid
- Myeloma.

Renal failure

Acute
- Abdominal plain X-ray (KUB) to exclude calculi.
- Ultrasound (US) is easy, immediate and accurate but it can be difficult to image obese patients.
- Radioisotope scanning to assess renal function.

Chronic
US to assess renal size and to exclude obstruction.

Computed tomography is useful to detect any extrinsic cause of obstruction.

Radioisotope scanning to assess treatment and prognosis.

Haematuria 1

Haematuria affects 10% of the general population. The signs and symptoms that may indicate its cause include:

- pain in the flank (trauma to the kidney, infection, stone or tumour)
- fever (infection of kidney or bladder)
- decreased urinary flow, hesitancy or incomplete voiding (lower urinary-tract obstruction, benign prostate hyperplasia or tumour)
- urinary urgency, pain or frequency (bladder cancer).

There are many different causes of haematuria (Box 1) and the clinical history, including the past history, age and ethnic background, and clinical examination should all be assessed before any imaging is performed. Some causes may require a urological (that is, surgical) intervention; some may stay under nephrological (that is, medical) management. In many situations, imaging is used to pick out the urological problems.

When presented with a patient with haematuria, the following basic information should be entered on the imaging request form:

- Painful or painless
- Gross or microscopic
- Continuous or transient.

The radiologist can then choose the imaging modality that will answer the diagnostic question most effectively.

A patient may attend with acute haematuria, but an intravenous urography (IVU) may not be the most appropriate first examination. As shown, most problems require more than one method of imaging. Adult patients will require cystoscopy to exclude small bladder tumours.

Painful gross haematuria

The patient may complain of flank pain and have a history of stones. In that case, an IVU is indicated to show the renal calculi (Fig. 1). Computed tomography (CT) may be needed to supplement this (Fig. 2).

Should the patient present with a mass, a renal tumour needs to be excluded (see pp 90–91). In this case, CT scanning is the primary method of investigation (Fig. 3), although a conventional IVU, plus ultrasound, would be a second best alternative.

Box 1 Causes of haematuria

Painful
- Calculi
- Infection
- If blood clots or flank pain – renal tumour.

Painless

Gross
- Bladder tumour
- Renal tumour
- Infection.

Microscopic
- Calculi
- Infection (possibly tuberculosis)
- Bladder tumour.

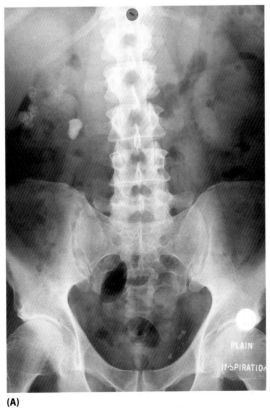
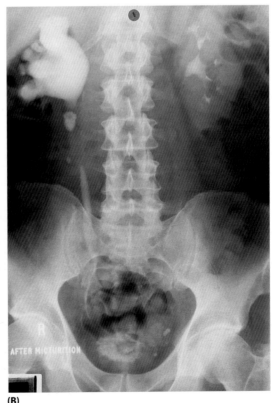

(A) **(B)**

Fig. 1 (A) **A plain abdominal X-ray (KUB)** demonstrating multiple small stones in the right kidney and a 2 cm stone possibly in the right ureter. (B) **Intravenous urography** confirms an obstructing ureteric stone.

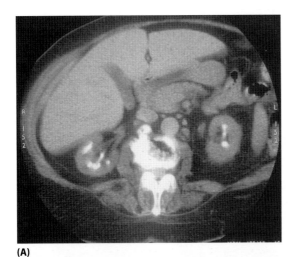

(A)

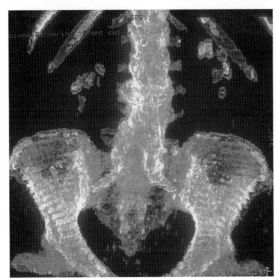

(B)

Fig. 2 (A) **A computed tomography (CT) scan** showing bilateral renal calculi. (B) **CT reconstruction** (volume rendering to remove soft tissue) showing the stones (and bones) in isolation.

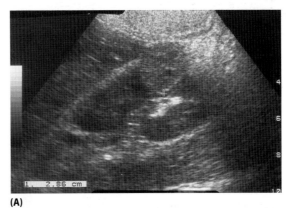

(A)

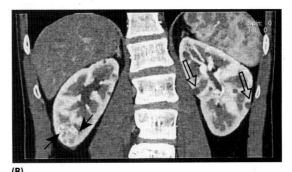

(B)

Fig. 3 (A) **The ultrasound shows a 3 cm solid echogenic (bright) mass** in the lower pole of the right kidney. (B) **Computed tomography examination following injection of contrast medium** with coronal reconstruction, confirms a renal tumour of the right kidney (closed arrows). Incidental simple cysts are shown (open arrows).

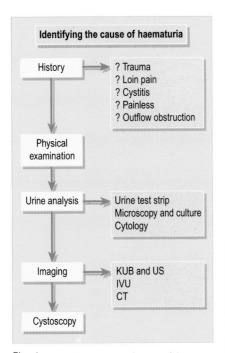

Identifying the cause of haematuria

History → ? Trauma
? Loin pain
? Cystitis
? Painless
? Outflow obstruction

Physical examination

Urine analysis → Urine test strip
Microscopy and culture
Cytology

Imaging → KUB and US
IVU
CT

Cystoscopy

Fig. 4 **Flow chart** for identification of the cause of haematuria.

Haematuria 1

- Intravenous urography (IVU) to show renal calculi, and exclude obstruction.

- Computed tomography (CT) if there is a renal mass especially in an elderly patient, alternatively IVU and ultrasound (US).

- IVU or US if a bladder tumour is suspected. Cystoscopy is indicated. IVU to exclude coexisting upper tract transitional cell carcinoma.

- US and IVU in a patient following prostatectomy.

- Plain abdominal X-ray (KUB) and US to exclude urinary tract infection in young female patient.

- IVU to exclude renal tuberculosis, papillary necrosis.

Haematuria 2

Painless haematuria

This is often related to a bladder tumour, for example, transitional cell carcinoma of the bladder (TCCB) (Fig. 1). An intravenous urography (IVU) would exclude a renal cause, while an ultrasound (US) of the bladder would demonstrate an obvious and large carcinoma. Cystoscopy would still be indicated. Where there is a history of bladder tumour, the upper tracts need careful follow-up as these also can develop transitional cell carcinoma (Fig. 2).

The patient may have had a previous transurethral prostatectomy (TURP). This procedure may result in bleeding from the prostatic bed and would present with painless haematuria, but it would still be necessary to exclude a renal cause for haematuria. Again, US and an IVU would be indicated.

Microscopic haematuria

If the patient is a young, fit female it is necessary to exclude urinary-tract infection, as well as stones. A plain film of the abdomen (KUB) should be obtained and an ultrasound to assess the upper renal tract for dilatation.

The bladder should be assessed before and after voiding to see how much residual urine remains. A large residual volume may predispose to infection and haematuria.

Occasionally infection, such as tuberculosis, may cause microscopic haematuria. Careful inspection of the renal calyces at IVU is necessary to exclude parenchymal destruction in this disease.

If patients have travelled to endemic areas, for instance, for schistosomiasis, the plain film should be inspected for bladder calcification, while US or IVU will also exclude upper renal-tract obstruction and stones.

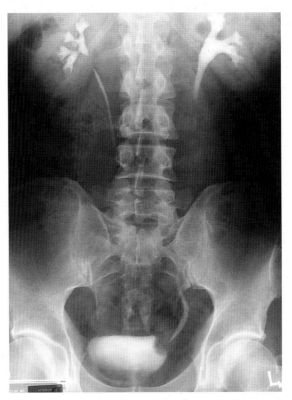

Fig. 1 **The full length intravenous urography demonstrates a small transitional cell carcinoma of the bladder** at the left ureteric orifice, which is not yet causing obstruction.

Table 1 **Investigation of renal trauma**		
	Blunt	**Penetrating**
Minor	US	US
Major	CT (? pedicle injury)	CT
Follow-up	Doppler US for renal blood flow	If evidence of direct vascular puncture –
	Radionuclide function study	angiography + ? segmental embolization

If intrinsic renal disease is suspected, a renal biopsy may subsequently be indicated.

Radiological investigation of renal trauma

Trauma can be divided into blunt flank trauma or penetrating trauma, as with a bullet or knife wound (Table 1). Minor blunt trauma with haematuria will only require US to see that there is no obvious extravasation of blood or urine collection. If haematuria persists, an IVU should exclude any underlying renal problem for the haematuria, such as a renal tumour.

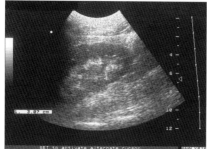

(A)

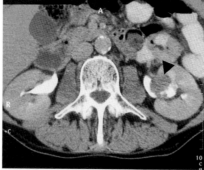

(C)

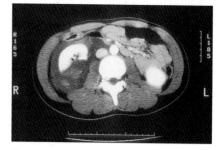

Fig. 3 **Trauma.** A computed tomography scan after contrast injection, showing a ruptured right kidney following a road-traffic accident; only the anterior half is opacified.

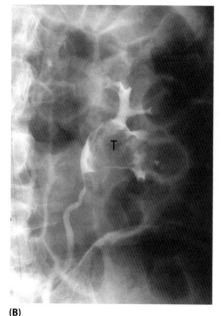

(B)

(D)

Fig. 2 **A patient presenting with gross painless haematuria**; previously treated for transitional cell carcinoma of the bladder. (A) At ultrasound a mass measuring 3 cm is detected in the left renal pelvis. (B) Intravenous urography confirms an irregular tumour (transitional cell carcinoma), but the computed tomography scans (C, D) show no evidence of the tumour invading the parenchyma.

Major blunt trauma, on the other hand, as with a deceleration road-traffic accident, may have resulted in trauma to the renal pedicle and requires an urgent computed tomography (CT) scan to ensure there has not been an avulsion injury to the renal vessels (Fig. 3). Even if there is no collection, such trauma to the renal vein may result in a renal vein thrombosis, and this must be followed carefully with colour Doppler ultrasound to check blood flow, and isotope renography to ensure normal renal function.

Haematuria 2

Renal trauma

■ There will be a history of trauma, followed by haematuria.

■ The plain film should be inspected for evidence of spinal or pelvic fractures.

■ Fractures of the transverse processes and ribs are associated with renal trauma.

■ Fractures of the pelvis are associated with bladder or urethral trauma.

■ The local soft tissues will be abnormal on the plain film.

■ The renal or bladder outlines may well be distorted.

■ Soft-tissue masses may be evident, especially in the pelvis, due to local haematomas.

■ Renal trauma may be seen on intravenous urography or at ultrasound, but is especially well seen at contrast-enhanced computed tomography (CT) scanning.

■ CT will also show bony trauma.

■ Ultrasound, including colour Doppler, shows anatomy and blood flow.

Renal masses

Investigation of renal masses

When a renal mass is found in the presence of haematuria, a renal tumour is of course suspected (Table 1), but a renal mass may be an incidental finding at an intravenous urography (IVU) or ultrasound (US) being performed for another reason.

The commonest mass is a simple renal cyst. Cysts are often extruded from the renal parenchyma, which has a marginal claw of soft tissue around the cyst. They can also displace the adjacent collecting system.

Renal cysts are generally smooth, round and well-defined. On an IVU, however, the mass effect of the cyst mimics a solid tumour. US will accurately differentiate the two. A simple cyst containing fluid will not attenuate the ultrasound and there will be no internal echoes; the mass will be 'anechoic'. A tumour on the other hand will nearly always have internal echoes from the tumour tissues. Very rarely, a very necrotic tumour that has a fluid centre will appear as a cyst. The wall is, however, usually irregular. If there are any doubts, a computed tomography (CT) scan before and after injection of intravenous contrast medium will show enhancement of a tumour (Fig. 1). Vascular tumours show enhancement with contrast medium; cysts do not. Solid tumours distort and compress the adjacent pelvicalyceal system (see also Box 1).

If a tumour is found at ultrasound, the renal vein and inferior vena cava (IVC) should be inspected to ensure that tumour thrombus is not extending into the IVC, which would alter the surgical approach (Fig. 2). The

Table 1 **Renal tumours**	
Benign	**Malignant**
Parenchymal	
Fibroma	Renal adenocarcinoma (renal cell carcinoma; hypernephroma)
Adenoma	Wilm's tumour (nephroblastoma)
Haemangioma (vascular tumour which can cause recurrent and profuse haematuria)	Sarcomas (rare)
Angiomyolipoma (common in tuberous sclerosis. Diagnosis made on CT, as fat easily visible within the tumour)	Secondaries from cancer., breast, bronchus, melanoma, lymphoma
Renal pelvis	
Papilloma	Transitional cell carcinoma (early presentation with haematuria or obstruction)
	Squamous cell carcinoma

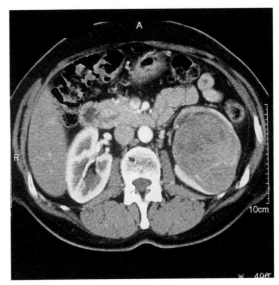

Fig. 1 **The computed tomography examination confirms a huge renal cell carcinoma** in the centre of the left kidney of this 60-year-old patient, who presented with gross haematuria and a left flank mass.

same applies at CT; however, this has the further advantage of demonstrating any extracapsular spread of tumour or enlargement of the peri-hilar lymph nodes.

Alternatively, magnetic resonance imaging (MRI) will show renal tumours and lymphadenopathy well (Fig. 3).

Tumours of the urogenital tract

Renal cell carcinoma (hypernephroma)

These lesions typically occur in males over 50 years of age and present with haematuria, loin pain and a mass. On occasion there may be hypertension or polycythaemia. The kidney is much expanded and distorted. There is a pathological circulation in the tumour. Survival is low, at 20%, if the renal vein

is involved early or if there is extension into the surrounding soft tissues.

Transitional cell carcinoma

This can occur anywhere in the lining of the urinary tract from the fornices of the calyces to the urethra, but is commonest in the bladder as urine is

Box 1 *Should a solid mass be biopsied?*

If positive – will have nephrectomy
If negative – still have nephrectomy (may have been missed on biopsy)
BUT
If lymphoma or metastatic disease suspected, biopsy may change management
Lymphoma – DXR or chemotherapy
Metastasis – treat primary first.

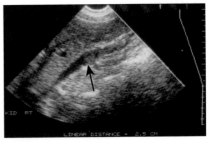

Fig. 2 **Longitudinal ultrasound of inferior vena cava** (IVC) behind the liver (arrow) with tumour thrombus in the IVC.

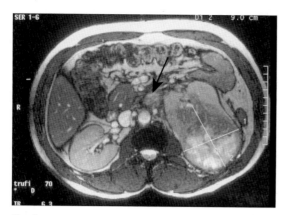

Fig. 3 **Magnetic resonance imaging** of left renal cell carcinoma (measured) with hilar nodal spread (arrow).

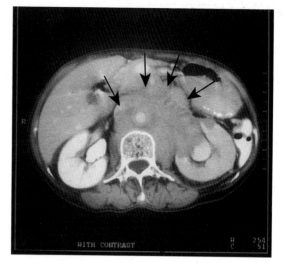

Fig. 4 **Lymphoma.** Computed tomography scan in a patient with huge retroperitoneal lymphadenopathy (arrows) due to lymphoma causing obstruction to the left kidney.

stored here, allowing the carcinogens in the urine a longer time to act on the bladder urothelium. Tumours in the pelvicalyceal system are rare, occasionally obstructing the pelvi-ureteric junction. Ureteric tumours are rarer still but, due to the narrow diameter of the ureter, will cause obstruction. A bladder tumour at a ureteric orifice may obstruct the entire upper tract (see Fig. 1).

Retrograde pyelography is rarely used today due to the excellent detail obtained by the IVU. Only occasionally is detail inadequate and retrograde catheterization is then requested to exclude small tumours.

Wilms' tumour (nephroblastoma)

This is the commonest intra-abdominal tumour in children, with a predominance between 1 and 4 years of age. The child presents with an abdominal mass, haematuria and intestinal obstruction. Widespread metastatic disease is often present when the child first attends.

These lesions are detected by ultrasound and, if large enough, will be seen on a plain film. The IVU will be grossly abnormal. CT scanning shows the lesion best, as well as local vascular and soft tissue invasion. Metastatic disease in the lungs is also assessed with CT scanning.

Sarcomas

Sarcomas are rare. Rhabdomyosarcoma of the bladder in young boys can give urinary obstruction.

Extrinsic tumours

Primary retroperitoneal tumours can obstruct the ureters by simple pressure effect (Fig. 4) or by direct ureteric invasion. Metastatic disease can act similarly by infiltrating the retroperitoneum and encasing the ureters.

In both these situations high-quality cross-sectional imaging is needed. Simple ultrasound will often diagnose the obstruction and identify a mass, but CT or MRI will be required to show more accurately the extent of the disease. Therefore, if the diagnosis is strongly suspected, the initial imaging should be with CT or MRI.

Renal masses

Tumours of the kidney
- Tumours of the kidney may be benign or malignant.
- The commonest benign mass lesion is the simple cyst.
- Cysts may be solitary or multiple, or may occur as an inherited disease – polycystic kidneys, sometimes in association with cystic change in other organs, e.g. liver and spleen.
- Being fluid-filled, cysts are transsonic at ultrasound examination and have a fluid attenuation at computed tomography (CT) and fluid signal at magnetic resonance imaging (MRI).
- Solid tumours may be benign or malignant.
- Malignant tumours have a pathological vascular supply, which is well demonstrated at ultrasound and with CT and MR angiography.
- Benign tumours displace the pelvicalyceal collecting system.
- Malignant tumours distort, infiltrate and invade the pelvicalyceal system.

Urinary-tract obstruction 1: causes

Urinary-tract obstruction can have a number of causes categorized as either congenital or aquired. Congenital causes include:

- pelvi-ureteric junction obstruction
- megaureter
- ureterocoele
- posterior urethral valves.

Acquired causes include:
- stones
- strictures
  - inflammatory: tuberculosis, retroperitoneal fibrosis
  - malignant: transitional cell carcinoma, extrinsic primary or secondary tumour
  - iatrogenic: damage at difficult pelvic surgery.

Congenital disorders causing urinary-tract obstruction

Pelvi-ureteric junction obstruction

This may be detected in utero at routine antenatal ultrasound, or present later in life if less severe. It can sometimes be demonstrated as an incidental finding at ultrasonography for non-specific pain.

Intravenous urography (IVU) is good for demonstrating the site of obstruction. If the diagnosis is suspected, but not initially apparent, a waterload and diuretic (frusemide) should be given at the time of the IVU (Fig. 1). If there is still doubt as to whether or not a pelvi-ureteric junction (PUJ) obstruction is present, radioisotope scanning using DTPA or MAG3, again followed by an intravenous injection of a diuretic, should be performed.

Obstruction due to a ureterocoele

The intra-mural portion of the ureter as it enters the bladder can be dilated (Fig. 2) and occasionally obstruct the upper tract.

Obstructed megaureter

An adynamic segment of ureter as it enters the bladder can give rise to upper tract obstruction and a dilated 'megaureter'.

Posterior urethral valves in boys

A valve in the posterior urethra may cause varying degrees of proximal distension of the urinary tract. This congenital abnormality may also be shown at routine antenatal ultrasound. The state of the kidneys in utero can also be assessed, as severe obstruction can lead to gross upper tract damage and renal failure.

Acquired causes of obstruction

Calculus disease

This is the commonest cause of acute renal obstruction.

A plain film of the abdomen and an ultrasound examination of the renal tract should be undertaken. These are simple and quick investigations. If a clear cut stone is seen, and the ultrasound shows a dilated renal tract, appropriate management can be instituted. A small stone, however, need not necessarily produce dilatation of the collecting system in the acute phase.

Ten per cent of stones are not opaque on X-ray. Small stones often arrest at the lower ureteric orifice, and these can be detected by an ultrasound scan through the abdominal wall with a full bladder.

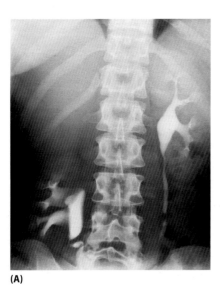

(A)

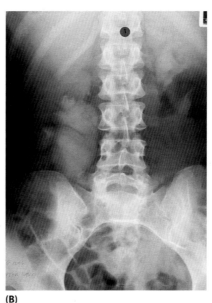

(B)

Fig. 1 **A patient with intermittent right flank pain after drinking.** (A) The 10-minute intravenous urograph shows floppy but apparently normal right kidney. (B) X-ray taken 10 minutes post Lasix diuretic. The left kidney contrast medium has washed out but the right kidney is dilated and obstructed at the PUJ.

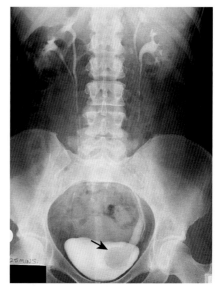

Fig. 2 **Intravenous urography.** Full length intravenous urography film with bilateral congenital duplication of the collecting systems and ureters. There is a non-obstructing ureterocoele on the left (arrow) (dilated intramural portion to the left ureter at the ureteric orifice).

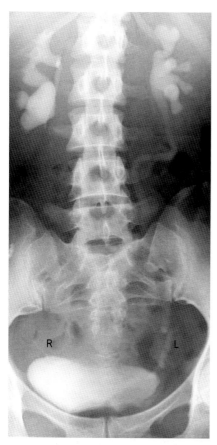

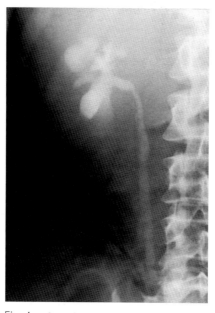

Fig. 4 **Tuberculosis.** Intravenous urography of right kidney showing dilated calyces and an irregular ureter due to tuberculosis.

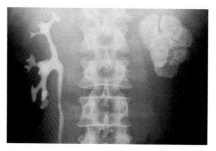

Fig. 5 **Previously untreated tuberculosis** has resulted in a calcified non-functioning left kidney (autonephrectomy).

Fig. 3 **Left ureteric obstruction due to carcinoma of the cervix** invading the bladder and obstructing the distal ureter. On the right there is a bifid calyceal system.

Malignant urinary-tract obstruction

In the elderly patient. the commonest cause of urinary-tract obstruction is malignancy (Fig. 3). This may cause obstruction by direct invasion of the ureters from a pelvic malignancy or due to the pressure effect of a large pelvic mass, or from encasement of the ureters in the retroperitoneum by lymph node metastases.

The upper tract obstruction may be detected by US but CT or MRI imaging is the best way to define the problem accurately. If the origin of the tumour is not apparent, US or CT-guided biopsy will be indicated.

Inflammatory causes of obstruction

Tuberculosis
Tuberculosis of the collecting system can cause stenosis of the calyces at the neck, and of the ureters at any level. Such strictures typically occur during treatment and healing.

If there is good function, intravenous urography (IVU) will detect obstruction

and also give fine detail of the calyces, detecting subtle changes of papillary erosions and calyceal distension (Fig. 4).

If function is impaired, a plain abdominal X-ray (KUB) is supplemented by ultrasound (US) examination. CT urography or magnetic resonance urography (MRU) may also be used in addition.

Untreated tuberculosis may lead to a non-functioning calcified kidney – a so-called *autonephrectomy* (Fig. 5).

Schistosomiasis (bilharzia; swimmer's itch)
S. haematobium is an infection with parasitic blood flukes (worms). This is found in much of equatorial and southern Africa, as well as in the north African countries bordering the Mediterranean. Inflammatory changes usually involve the ureters and bladder with haematuria.

The plain film may show characteristic bladder calcification, which is due to large numbers of calcified eggs in the bladder wall (Fig. 6). Calcification is better shown on CT.

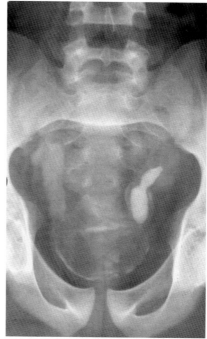

Fig. 6 **Schistosomiasis.** There is calcification of the bladder wall and dilatation of the lower ureters. The distended ureteric walls are also calcified and, on the left, a large lower ureteric calculus is shown. An intravenous urograph will show renal parenchymal damage, lower ureteric obstruction and dilatation.

Calcification is better shown at computed tomography than on a plain film.

Renal damage with hydronephrosis may be the end result of urinary-tract outflow obstruction.

Sexually transmitted diseases
Pelvic tumours can obstruct the ureter either by pressure effect or by direct involvement of the ureter.

Urinary-tract obstruction 1: causes

Acute
- Plain abdominal X-ray (KUB) and ultrasound (US) – simple, but poor specificity.
- Intravenous urography – good at demonstrating site of obstruction.
- Computed tomography (CT) – rapid diagnosis, high sensitivity.

Chronic
- US – dilated kidneys; may pick up extrinsic mass.
- CT or magnetic resonance imaging – best definition for retroperitoneum.

Urinary-tract obstruction 2: radiological investigations

Emergency intravenous urography

This examination is limited to detect obstruction, not to give detailed images of the urinary tract. A plain film is taken, the intravenous contrast medium is injected, and then a film of the abdomen obtained at 15 minutes. There may be a prolonged nephrogram, with persistent opacification of the renal parenchyma, and delay in contrast medium reaching the collecting system.

Later films at 1 hour, 4 hours and, sometimes, 12 hours will then be necessary to allow the trapped contrast medium to filter down to confirm a ureteric obstruction by a stone (Fig. 1).

Ultrasound

Often, in an acute colic, the patient has a previous history of calculus disease. If, in this situation, a KUB has shown an opacity near the pelvi-ureteric or uretero-vesical junction, a simple ultrasound may confirm a urinary tract stone. The renal pelvic stone can be seen related to the renal outline; a stone at the uretero-vesical junction can be detected by scanning through a full bladder. In addition US may show some dilatation of the underlying kidney confirming obstruction as the cause for pain. An IVU can thus be avoided.

If the opacity is in the line of the ureter, it may be impossible to pick it up on US. A limited IVU may therefore be indicated.

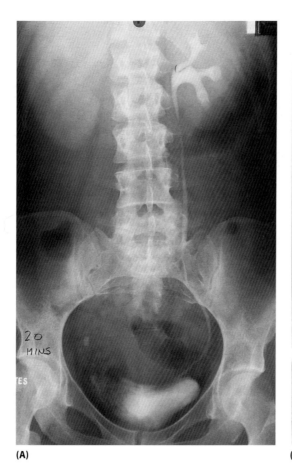
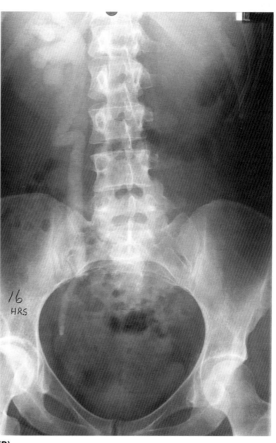

(A) (B)

Fig. 1 **A 40-year-old woman with right renal colic.** The plain film showed a suspected right ureteric stone. (A) The 20-minute intravenous urograph shows delayed excretion on the right. (B) The late film confirms a stone obstructing the right ureter.

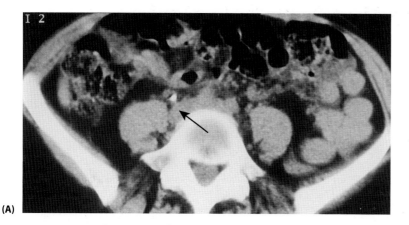

(A)

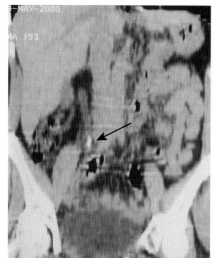

(B)

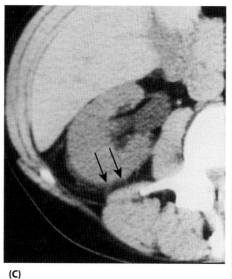

(C)

Computed tomography

A very rapid computed tomography (CT) examination can be obtained without any preparation or intravenous contrast medium. This has the great advantage of rapid diagnosis. All stones can be detected (Fig. 2). Ureteric dilatation can also be shown. Unfortunately, occasionally pelvic phleboliths may be misdiagnosed as calculi.

Urinary-tract obstruction 2: radiological investigations

Tuberculosis
- Intravenous urography if good function.
- Plain abdominal X-ray (KUB) and ultrasound if impaired function.
- Can also use computed tomography (CT) urography or magnetic resonance urography.

Schistosomiasis
- KUB or CT.

Sexually transmitted diseases
- Urethrography for urethral strictures.

Imaging malignant obstruction

US
- Dilated upper tracts.

CT/MRI
- Lymphoma.
- Metastatic breast cancer.

Fig. 2 (A) **Spiral non-contrast computed tomography** rapidly confirms a right ureteric stone as the cause for colic. (B) **Coronal reconstruction** showing a dilated right ureter above the stone (arrow). (C) **Computed tomography of right kidney.** The obstruction causes peri-renal oedema – a secondary sign of obstruction – seen as fibrous stranding (arrows).

Lower urinary tract

Lower urinary-tract symptoms (LUTS) is an all-embracing term used by urologists covering bladder and urethral symptoms from mild urinary frequency, irritation and dysuria, to obstruction and incontinence: all these symptoms can be due to multiple causes (see Boxes 1 & 2 for appropriate investigations). The most useful imaging technique in these cases is ultrasound (US) of the bladder combined with measurement of urinary flow rates (Fig. 1) and a post-micturition US of residual urine volumes.

Box 1 Investigation of lower urinary tract symptoms

History
Physical examination
Urinalysis
- Haematuria
- Infection
- Cytology
Imaging
- Bladder ultrasound (US)
- Urine flow rate
- US of residual urine
- Intravenous urography if stones, transitional cell carcinoma or tuberculosis suspected
Uro-dynamic pressure/flow test: to show obstruction or instability.

Box 2 Radiological investigation of the lower urinary tract

Lower urinary-tract symptoms
- Ultrasound (US) bladder and measurement of urinary flow rates
- Post-micturition US of residual urine volumes
Urinary-tract infection
- US kidney
- Post-micturition US of residual urine volumes
Stones
- Plain abdominal X-ray (KUB)
- Intravenous urography (IVU)
Transitional cell carcinoma
- IVU to exclude upper tract involvement
Tuberculosis
- IVU
Prostatic carcinoma
- Transrectal ultrasound
- US-guided biopsy
Urethral valves
- Prenatal US
- Descending micturating urethrogram
Urethral strictures
- Ascending urethrogram
Trauma
- Ascending urethrogram to show anterior ureter
- Descending urethrogram to show posterior ureter.

Causes of lower urinary-tract symptoms

Urinary-tract infection
Recurrent urinary tract infection (UTI) will give urinary frequency and dysuria. Underlying anatomical abnormalities need to be excluded. The main cause of recurrent infection is failure to empty the bladder at micturition.

Stones
Lower ureteric calculi and bladder calculi will irritate the lower urinary tract resulting in frequency.

Transitional cell carcinoma
Transitional cell carcinoma (TCC) of the bladder can present with urinary frequency as well as haematuria (see p. 88). The required investigations in suspected bladder tumour are:

- urinalysis
- cytology
- cystoscopy.

While imaging is not important in the *diagnosis* of bladder tumours, its role is to exclude involvement of the upper urinary tracts, as TCC can occur anywhere in the lining of the urinary tract. Intravenous urography (IVU) is the imaging of choice.

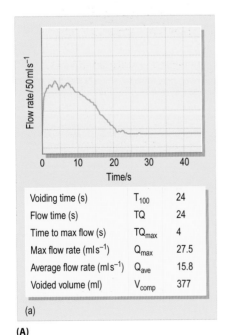

Voiding time (s)	T_{100}	24
Flow time (s)	TQ	24
Time to max flow (s)	TQ_{max}	4
Max flow rate (ml s^{-1})	Q_{max}	27.5
Average flow rate (ml s^{-1})	Q_{ave}	15.8
Voided volume (ml)	V_{comp}	377

(a)

(A)

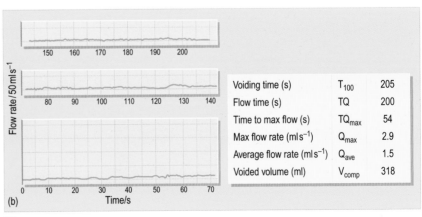

Voiding time (s)	T_{100}	205
Flow time (s)	TQ	200
Time to max flow (s)	TQ_{max}	54
Max flow rate (ml s^{-1})	Q_{max}	2.9
Average flow rate (ml s^{-1})	Q_{ave}	1.5
Voided volume (ml)	V_{comp}	318

(b)

(B)

Fig. 1 **(A) Normal flow rate. (B) Grossly delayed flow rate.**

Tuberculosis

Tuberculosis may give frequency and dysuria. An IVU should be performed.

Interstitial cystitis

This may produce severe frequency and dysuria. Other causes need to be excluded. The diagnosis is made at cystoscopy.

Bladder instability

Abnormal unstable bladder contractions can be a cause of urgency and require specialized lower-tract urodynamic assessment with fine bladder pressure catheters.

Imaging of the prostate

Benign enlargement of the prostate itself is unimportant and requires no imaging. If there are secondary symptoms to suggest lower-tract obstruction, then imaging for LUTS as above is indicated.

Tumours of the prostate

A tumour of the prostate gland can be suspected at digital examination of the prostate (DRE), when the prostate-specific antigen (PSA) blood test is elevated or when a transrectal ultrasound examination (TRUS) detects an area of low echogenicity (Figs 2 & 3).

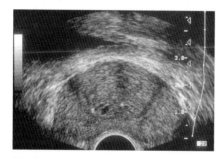

Fig. 2 **Transaxial TRUS of normal prostate.**

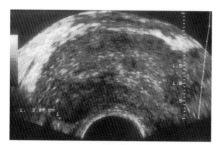

Fig. 3 **TRUS with carcinoma**, seen as low echogenic (dark) area in the right peripheral zone (measured).

With the increasing use of the PSA blood test to screen for suspected carcinoma, clinicians are requesting confirmation by biopsy of the prostate. This is best done under US guidance. A transrectal US probe with biopsy attachment allows accurate biopsies to be taken, concentrating on the peripheral zone of the gland where 70–80% of tumours originate.

Currently, biopsies are taken when any of the three tests are suspicious (DRE, PSA or US).

Imaging of the urethra

Urethral valves

Posterior urethral valves are the main congenital abnormalities in boys. If severe, they may be detected in utero, with upper-tract obstruction and gross hydronephrosis at pre-natal US.

In the infant, a descending micturating urethrogram will fill out the valves like a sail. This requires gentle catheterization in order to first fill the bladder with contrast medium.

Urethral strictures

These are usually acquired either by gonococcal or tuberculous infection, or iatrogenic from irritation due to a catheter. These are best shown by an ascending urethrogram injecting contrast medium via a clamp or catheter to outline the penile and bulbar urethra.

Trauma

This may result in gross disruption of the urethra, requiring complicated surgery.

In an acute injury with bleeding per urethra, a catheter should not be passed; if necessary, a suprapubic catheter is placed. A gentle ascending urethrogram may clear the urethra to allow passage of a catheter.

Severe disruption of the urethra is difficult to repair and is usually left to settle with a suprapubic catheter. Later, ascending and descending studies will be needed to plan subsequent reconstruction (Fig. 4).

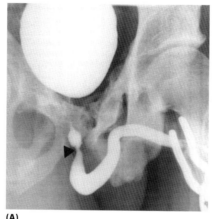

(A)

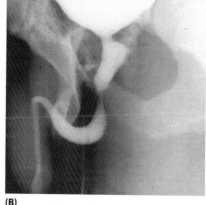

(B)

Fig. 4 (A) **Ascending urethrogram** with tight stricture (arrow) following fractured pelvis. Note irregular pubic bones. (B) **Descending study** confirming a normal wide posterior urethra above the stricture.

Lower urinary tract

Bladder cancer
- Not diagnosed by imaging – needs cystoscopy
- Can be multifocal, therefore, needs intravenous urography to clear upper tract.

Lower urinary-tract symptoms
- Ultrasound and flow rates first
- Remember can be due to:
  - Stones
  - Transitional cell carcinoma
  - Tuberculosis.

Central Nervous System

Imaging techniques in neuroradiology 1

Computed tomography

Computed tomography (CT) is an X-ray investigation producing sectional images, usually in the axial plane. As the information acquired is digital, it can, for instance, be manipulated to produce images optimized for bone as well as for soft tissues. With the latest generation equipment, sub-second scans are produced resulting in very short examination times.

Cranial CT is the imaging method of choice for spontaneous and traumatic acute cerebral bleeds. The patient is supine, it is quick, simple to perform and its ability to demonstrate intracranial haemorrhage determines its first-line status in stroke. A mass lesion, due either to haemorrhage or to a tumour causing raised intracranial pressure, will also be readily apparent.

Trauma is a particularly good example of the versatility of CT where, besides obtaining the cerebral images, it is possible to examine the skull vault and base for fracture (Fig. 1). In severe trauma, the examination can be extended to include the vertebral column, chest, abdomen, pelvis and limbs as necessary.

Magnetic resonance imaging

Magnetic resonance imaging (MRI) is the mainstay of cranial and spinal imaging in adults and children. Its ability to delineate cerebral pathology, particularly white-matter disease, is generally far superior to CT. There are exceptions, however. Haemorrhage and bony anatomy are better imaged with CT and, allied to this, CT is much more sensitive to the presence of calcification in a lesion than MRI. This can be useful in tumour diagnosis and, in many instances, patients will have both CT and MRI.

MRI is concerned with protons, which are well represented in water and fat, and thus in soft tissue but not in bone. With the patient in a powerful magnetic field, protons are energized by a transient radiofrequency pulse and then allowed to 'relax' or return to their resting state, emitting energy in so doing. There are various ways both

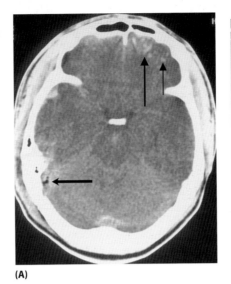 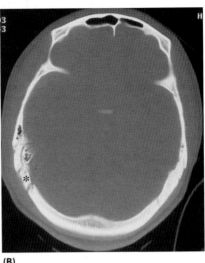

(A) **(B)**

Fig. 1 **Severe trauma – cranial computed tomography (CT).** The same CT slice (A) on soft-tissue windows showing contusions (arrows) and (B) on bone windows revealing a fracture complex (*) not visible on (A). Locules of air are also seen in (A), indicating that this is a compound fracture (horizontal arrow).

to apply the radiofrequency pulses and to measure relaxation. This results in a number of 'pulse sequences', which yield a corresponding variety of images.

Broadly, T1-weighted images demonstrate anatomy and any enhancement following an intravenous injection of the MR contrast agent, gadolinium DTPA; T2-weighted images show cerebral parenchymal change well. There are many more pulse sequences, however, each with particular advantages. As a result of the multiple sequences even in a routine study, MRI scans take longer to complete than CT, which is a further reason for the preferred use of the latter in the emergency situation.

The representation of haemorrhage on MRI is complex because the different forms of haemoglobin each

have different 'signal characteristics'. In addition, whereas haemorrhage disappears after 1 or 2 weeks on CT, on MRI the evidence can be present, in some cases, indefinitely. One can follow the evolution of a haematoma and often decide whether multiple haematomas are of different ages (Table 1). This is especially valuable in non-accidental injury in children, when evidence of repeated trauma is crucial.

Diffusion weighted MRI (DWI) is finding an important role in the diagnosis of early cerebral infarction, particularly in the presence of chronic ischaemia. As its name implies, in DWI the appearances are based on the diffusion of protons in water. This will be unimpeded in, for example, cerebrospinal fluid, but restricted in early infarction (Fig. 2).

Table 1 **The evolution of haemorrhage on magnetic resonance imaging**			
		T1	T2
Hyperacute (2–3 hours)	Oxyhaemoglobin	Dark	Bright
Acute (up to 4 days)	Deoxyhaemoglobin	Isointense	Dark
Subacute: (4–7 days)	Methaemoglobin	Bright	Dark
Subacute: (6 days –8 weeks)	Methaemoglobin	Bright	Bright
Chronic (8 weeks onwards)	Haemosiderin	Isointense	Dark
(Adapted from Hadley DM, Teasdale EM 2000 In: Gillespie JE, Jackson A (eds) MRI and CT of the brain. Arnold, London, p. 86).			

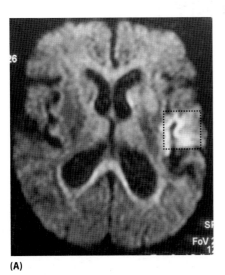
(A)

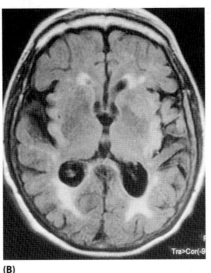
(B)

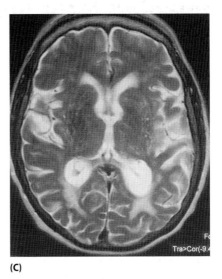
(C)

Fig. 2 **Acute on chronic cerebral ischaemia in a patient presenting with acute dysphasia.** (A) The diffusion weighted magnetic resonance (MR) image clearly demonstrates acute ischaemia in the posterior sylvian region. (B) The T2-weighted and (C) FLAIR MR images at the same level fail to disclose any definite acute change. The confluent high signal in white matter and the punctate basal ganglia lesions are due to chronic 'small vessel' ischaemia.

MRI in the investigation of spinal disease

In spinal disease, the facility to undertake sagittal surveillance, where multilevel disease is suspected (for example, metastases) or in cases where the level is unclear, utilizes the inherent multiplanar facility of MRI. MR images can be produced in any plane, although the axial, sagittal and coronal (the orthogonal) planes are the norm.

MRI is the investigation of choice for intervertebral discal disease (see p. 14) and is the only method to image the spinal cord directly (Fig. 3). Bone is not imaged directly because of the paucity of free protons in calcium. Dense cortical bone is represented as a region of 'signal void' (black). The signal from vertebral bodies derives from the bone marrow (yellow or fatty in adults, red or haematopoietic in children). Subtle changes to the signal, as can occur in neoplastic infiltration, make MRI extremely sensitive to vertebral involvement in metastatic disease.

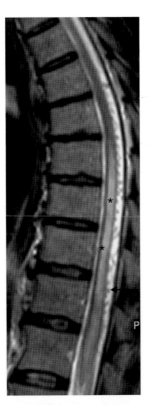

Fig. 3 **Spinal arteriovenous malformation.** The sagittal T2-weighted MR image of the thoracic spine shows oedema within the spinal cord (*). The irregular shapes seen immediately posterior to the cord are the abnormal vessels (arrow).

Imaging techniques in neuroradiology 1

■ Computed tomography is the initial investigation of choice for suspected acute intracranial haemorrhage and in stroke.

■ Magnetic resonance imaging is much more sensitive to cerebral parenchymal change and is the preferred investigation in the majority of non-emergency situations.

■ T1-weighted MRI sequences demonstrate anatomy well.

■ T2-weighted MRI sequences are more sensitive to cerebral parenchymal pathology.

■ Changes due to haemorrhage resolve rapidly (over days) with CT, but can persist for months or years with MRI.

Imaging techniques in neuroradiology 2

Angiography

The selective injection of iodinated contrast agent into the cervical vessels through a catheter inserted into the carotid and vertebral arteries (and sometimes the internal jugular veins) remains the gold standard for cerebral angiography. Modern angiography utilizes digital subtraction techniques (DSA), where the bone and soft-tissue detail are 'removed' from the image leaving the craniocervical vasculature in isolation (Fig. 1). Microcatheters and microguidewires inserted through the larger catheters form the basis of interventional (therapeutic) neuroradiology.

Less invasive or non-invasive methods are challenging DSA in diagnosis. Computed tomography angiography (CTA), using the new multislice CT scanners, necessitates an intravenous injection of iodinated contrast medium. Magnetic resonance angiography (MRA) can be performed with or without intravenous gadolinium DTPA.

A further development in DSA is rotational angiography, where the

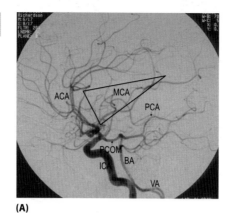

(A)

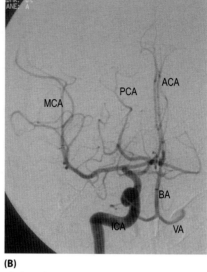

(B)

Fig. 1 **Normal study – internal carotid arterial DSA.** (A) Lateral and (B) frontal projections. With a single projection, the 3-D orientation of these arteries may not be appreciated. Note that the ACAs run near to the midline, the MCA branches laterally and the PCAs posteriorly. In (A) the proximal MCA branches are within the triangle.

ACA, anterior cerebral arteries; BA, basilar artery; ICA, internal carotid artery; MCA, middle cerebral artery; PCA, posterior cerebral artery; PCOM, posterior communicating artery; VA, vertebral artery (paired).

X-ray tube and detector rotate in an arc. The derived data can be used to produce 3-D images (3-D angiography), which like CTA and MRA, are digital images, which can be manipulated on a workstation and viewed from any direction.

Ultrasonography

Duplex carotid ultrasonography is a valuable screening method in suspected cervical carotid artery stenosis (Fig. 2). Atherosclerosis, depending on the severity and nature

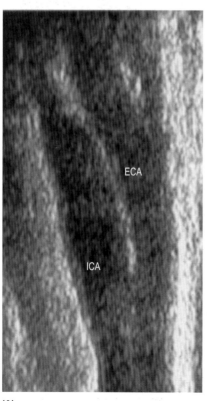

(A)

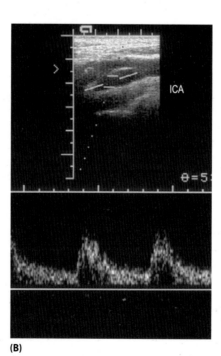

(B)

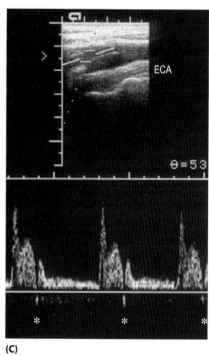

(C)

Fig. 2 **Normal examination – duplex carotid sonography.** (A) The B mode study shows the larger internal carotid artery (ICA) and the external carotid artery (ECA), which branches in the neck. (B and C) **Doppler studies.** Velocity is on the y axis, time on the x. The ICA trace is shown in (B), typical of a circulation with low total peripheral resistance with blood flow continuing throughout the cardiac cycle. The ECA trace reflects the high total peripheral resistance of the craniofacial arteries, where blood flow ceases or even reverses in diastole (*).

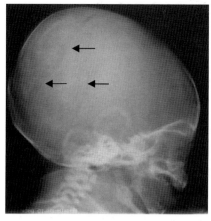

Fig. 3 **Lateral skull radiograph in a baby with suspected non-accidental injury.** There are bilateral parietal fractures. The wide separation of one fracture is suspicious but the final diagnosis is reached after rigorous clinical, radiological, social and, ultimately, judicial assessments.

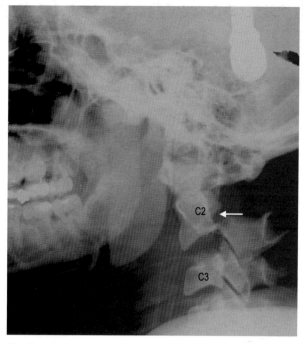

Fig. 4 **Hangman's fracture of the second cervical vertebra (the axis, C2).** There has been a fracture through the pedicles (arrow). This is the injury said to be caused by judicial (not suicidal) hanging.

of the 'plaque' in this region can be a risk factor for stroke. The 'B mode' element of the examination shows the atherosclerotic deposits or plaque on the vessel wall; the Doppler study measures the velocity of blood in the region of the cervical carotid bifurcation. In excess of 50% diameter stenosis, the velocity increases in proportion to the degree of stenosis.

Plain radiography

Radiography of the skull in non-traumatic cerebral disease is rarely performed since it contributes little, if anything, to diagnosis. It may be obtained before or after cranial surgery for specific indications. Even in trauma, its role is controversial, with the notable exception of suspected child abuse, where the type of fracture can be important (Fig. 3). The controversy in trauma stems from the large number of normal studies obtained and the fact that it is the status of the intracranial contents which is of primary interest. To some extent CT sidesteps the dilemma, permitting both skull and brain to be studied. Of course fractures of the vault parallel to the scan plane can be overlooked, but CT is undoubtedly superior for skull-base fractures and the preliminary step in all cranial CT exams is the acquisition of a lateral digital radiograph of the skull, so that the slices can be positioned.

Radiography of the vertebral column is usually obtained following trauma (Fig. 4). It provides rapid sagittal surveillance, which is not readily obtained using CT, even with digital localizers. CT, confined to axial scanning, can thus be directed to specific regions of interest, showing often complex fractures in detail (Fig. 5).

Lateral radiographs are also a simple means of assessing the vertebral alignment and mobility of the spinal column with views obtained in flexion and extension.

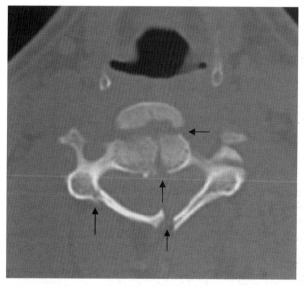

Fig. 5 **Complex cervical fracture.** The axial CT shows multiple fractures (arrows). Note the foramen transversarium which transmits the vertebral arteries. These are at risk in severe cervical trauma.

Imaging techniques in neuroradiology 2

- Carotid and vertebral angiography remains the gold standard to demonstrate the intracranial blood vessels.

- Non-invasive techniques currently used, however, include computed tomography angiography (to demonstrate the blood vessels following intravenous injection of iodinated contrast medium into the arm) and magnetic resonance angiography, which demonstrates the cerebral circulation, with or without the intravenous injection of gadolinium.

- Ultrasound is a commonly used screening technique to identify atheromatous disease of the carotid arteries and the severity of any narrowing on the blood flow.

- Plain radiography is of limited value in the investigation of intracranial pathology.

Imaging techniques in neuroradiology 3

Myelography

Myelography is an invasive investigation of the spinal contents, which has largely been replaced by magnetic resonance imaging (MRI). Iodinated contrast medium is injected into the spinal subarachnoid space by lumbar or cervical needle puncture to outline the nerve roots and spinal cord. The procedure is usually supplemented by computed tomography (CT) (CT myelography). Currently, myelography is usually reserved for patients who are intolerant of MRI (claustrophobia being a recognized problem) or in whom MRI is contraindicated (cardiac pacemaker, cochlear implant, etc.). Myelography may also be required in patients with suspected neural compression after the insertion of metallic spinal surgical implants. While posing no inherent danger to the patient undergoing MRI or CT, the implants may cause severe degradation of the image.

Cisternography

Iodinated contrast medium introduced via lumbar puncture can be made to

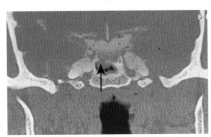

(A)

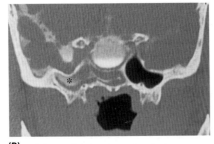

(B)

Fig. 1 **CT cisternogram.** These coronal scans show a defect in the floor of the pituitary fossa (arrow) (A). Contrast medium (*) has entered the sphenoid sinus, which is not aerated due to trans-sphenoidal surgery to remove a pituitary tumour (B).

enter the cranial subarachnoid space by careful positioning of the patient. It is used to identify the site of leakage of cerebrospinal fluid (CSF) through a tear in the dural lining of the skull base due to either trauma or surgery (Fig. 1). The condition may also develop spontaneously and can lead to CSF leakage through the nose (CSF rhinorrhoea) or ear (CSF otorrhoea).

For a successful study the patient should be actively leaking and, if preliminary CT clearly shows a bone defect in an appropriate position, cisternography may be unnecessary.

The condition should be suspected when patients develop recurrent meningitis.

Magnetic resonance spectroscopy

While MR imaging uses the magnetic properties of protons in water to create images, there are many protons in other molecules that do not contribute to the image. These protons are present in tiny amounts compared to those in water, but many are in compounds that are of considerable interest to clinicians and researchers. Although it is not possible to create anatomical images from these compounds, MR spectroscopy can measure their relative concentration within living tissue, and present these concentrations as a spectrum (Fig. 2). Within the brain, several useful compounds can be measured, leading to an accurate measure of the metabolic activity within the volume of interest. Of the more important compounds, N-Acetyl Aspartate (NAA) gives an indication of the number of viable neurons and axons present, and is significantly reduced, for example, in infarction; choline is a measure of cell membrane turnover, and is commonly elevated in tumours such as glioma. Lactate can be demonstrated in a number of pathological states where there is a failure of normal aerobic metabolism. MR spectroscopy is now commonly being used in clinical practice as an adjunct to MRI to assess the degree of malignancy in cerebral tumours, and to refine the specificity of MRI in patients with white-matter disorders.

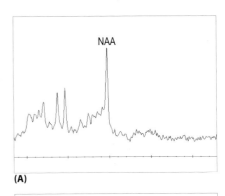

(A)

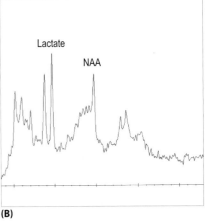

(B)

Fig. 2 (A) **Normal spectrum**: note the large central peak of NAA, representing normal neurons and axons. (B) **Abnormal spectrum from a child with a brain infarct**: the NAA peak is greatly reduced, and there is a new abnormal peak representing lactate. (With kind permission of Dr Shawn Halpin, Consultant Neuroradiologist, University Hospital of Wales, Cardiff.)

Positron emission tomography

Positron emission tomography (PET) scanning combines radioisotopes with relatively short half-lives with fairly accurate spatial localization of any lesion. The commonest radiopharmaceutical in routine use is ^{18}Fluorodeoxyglucose, which is incorporated into the glycolytic cycle and 'trapped'. Metabolically active, neoplastic cells are thus identified and PET, among a variety of applications, has proved valuable in distinguishing cerebral tumour recurrence (metabolically active) from post-irradiation changes (metabolically inactive), which can look identical on MRI scans (Fig. 3). PET is now co-located with CT in the same 'scanner' as PET-CT.

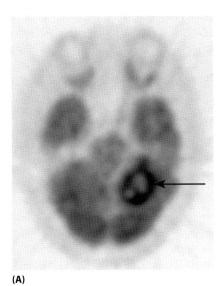

(A)

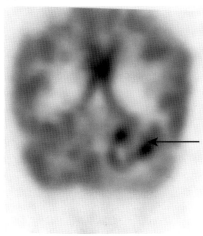

(B)

Fig. 3 **An ¹⁸FDG PET scan showing recurrence of a metastasis from carcinoma of the colon** (arrow) after surgical resection and post-operative radiotherapy. (A) axial and (B) coronal images.

Guidelines to imaging in neurological disease

From the above it will be clear that there may be several approaches to a particular problem, determined by the patient's condition and, to some extent, local availability of both scanners and expertise. In many cases the patient may undergo multiple complementary investigations.

Cranial emergencies

In the *emergency situation*, strategies must be devised to identify reliably those conditions requiring urgent

treatment and, once these have been ruled out, then evaluation can occur at a more leisurely pace. Of course, in general the prime determinant of any imaging strategy will be the clinical picture.

Thus, cranial CT is the initial investigation of choice in the majority of cranial emergencies; in the **unconscious patient**, when a cerebral cause is possible, in the patient with suspected **stroke** or **intracranial haemorrhage** and in **head injury**.

The patient with **raised intracranial pressure**, depending on its severity, may be imaged initially with CT or MRI. It may of course be a consequence of any of the conditions above, but should there be an **intracranial tumour** or **intracranial abscess** then MRI will almost always be undertaken as part of surgical planning.

MRI will also be used when a posterior fossa infarct is suspected, because of the comparative insensitivity of CT in abnormalities in this location.

The subsequent imaging investigation of stroke will usually involve some form of angiography of the cervical arteries, increasingly MRA or CTA rather than catheter angiography. In the investigation of **subarachnoid and intraparenchymal haemorrhage**, the less invasive methods are also gaining popularity, although catheter angiography remains the gold standard.

An epileptic seizure, without resultant trauma, in a known epileptic patient does not necessarily require imaging evaluation. Cranial CT is also not regarded as an essential

prerequisite to diagnostic lumbar puncture.

Spinal disorders

In **spinal trauma**, plain film studies followed by CT are undertaken. The association of cranial and spinal injury is well known and, in severe cases with an unconscious patient, a combined CT study may be performed. MRI in trauma is valuable to examine the spinal soft tissues, notably, the spinal cord for contusion or haemorrhage, the ligaments and intervertebral discs.

In non-traumatic **spinal cord or nerve root compression**, MRI is the preferred investigation. Plain radiography is unrewarding in patients with backache and sciatica.

Non-emergency ('outpatient') setting

Common neurological symptoms such as chronic headache, dizziness or deafness are investigated using MRI, in the majority of cases, to rule out a serious structural abnormality. If the headache and facial pain are thought to be due to paranasal sinus disease, then CT may be preferred.

Transient ischaemic attacks (TIAs) are often investigated with duplex sonography in combination with MRI or CT. It is, however, perfectly acceptable to use cranial CT and cervical CTA or MRI and MRA.

Suspected congenital anomalies of the brain or spinal cord and all types of epilepsy are best analysed using MRI.

Acknowledgement

The section on magnetic resonance spectroscopy was contributed by Dr Shawn Halpin, Consultant Neuroradiologist, University Hospital of Wales, Cardiff.

Imaging techniques in neuroradiology 3

- Magnetic resonance imaging is the investigation of choice for pathology affecting the vertebral column, spinal cord and nerve roots.

- Myelography (the injection of iodinated contrast medium into the subarachnoid space) is usually reserved for those patients who are unable to undergo MRI and is performed infrequently. It is usually supplemented by CT scanning (CT myelography).

- Positron emission tomography can be used to distinguish recurrent cerebral tumours from the effects of radiotherapy. It has other applications in tumour diagnosis elsewhere in the body.

Ischaemic stroke

Stroke is defined as the sudden onset of a focal neurological deficit, of presumed vascular origin, classically lasting in excess of 24 hours. With the necessity for thrombolytic therapy to be instituted early, ideally within 3 hours, the time element in the definition is now less clear.

The majority of strokes are ischaemic and usually result from thromboembolic disease originating at the cervical carotid arterial bifurcation, a favoured site for atherosclerosis. The heart is also a potential source of emboli, particularly from thrombus within a poorly contracting and ischaemic left ventricle. Cerebral haemorrhage is the second commonest cause of stroke and, rarely, cerebral tumours may be responsible even in the absence of intratumoral haemorrhage.

Imaging of the stroke patient

The commonest manifestation of stroke is the sudden onset of hemiparesis due to middle-cerebral or internal-carotid artery occlusion, but a variety of clinical syndromes exist, depending on the vascular territory involved. Computed tomography (CT) in infarction will show low density due to increased water content in the appropriate vascular territory (Figs 1 & 2), but may be normal for the first 24 hours. Infarction due to basilar artery thrombosis may lead to oedema of the cerebellum, obstruction of the fourth ventricle and hydrocephalus, constituting a neurosurgical emergency (Fig. 3). It is also the case that ischaemia can result from disease in the small intracranial arteries, which affects the less well vascularized white matter, producing so-called angiopathic or small vessel ischaemic change (Fig. 4). Magnetic resonance imaging (MRI) is valuable, particularly with the more subtle lesions in the posterior fossa and for its angiographic capability.

Haemorrhagic infarcts
Haemorrhagic infarcts occur when there is dissolution of an embolus and reperfusion of the ischaemic region. Such haemorrhagic conversion usually occurs after the initial ischaemic event and may be heralded by further clinical deterioration.

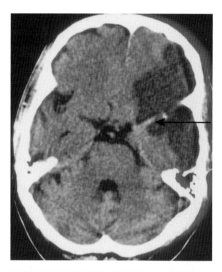

Fig. 1 **Infarct.** A cranial computed tomography scan showing the middle cerebral artery. Note the hyperdense, thrombosed middle cerebral artery (arrow).

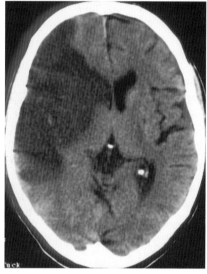

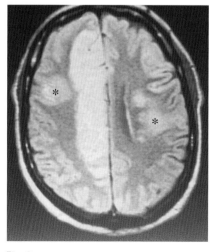

Fig. 2 **Multiple cerebral emboli.** The cranial magnetic resonance image shows right anterior cerebral artery infarction in the typical paramedian 'Mohican' distribution. There are also bilateral middle cerebral artery infarctions (*).

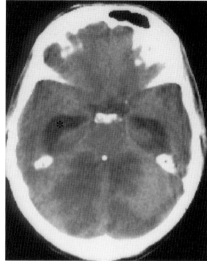

Fig. 3 **Cerebellar infarction** due to basilar artery thrombosis is demonstrated on this cranial computed tomography scan as an area of low attenuation (dark) change in the cerebellum. Note the enlarged inferior (temporal) horns of the lateral ventricle (*).

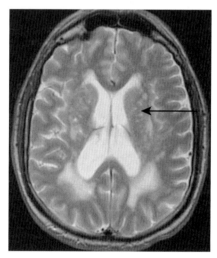

Fig. 4 **Small vessel ischaemic change.** A combination of punctate and confluent lesions in the periventricular white matter and within the basal ganglia (arrow) is shown on a cranial magnetic resonance image.

Dissection of the cervical carotid or vertebral arteries
An increasingly recognized cause of cerebral ischaemia is dissection of the cervical carotid or vertebral arteries, which may occur after minor trauma or, indeed, apparently spontaneously (Fig. 5). The clinical association of cerebral ischaemia following cervical pain in a young adult is an important clue.

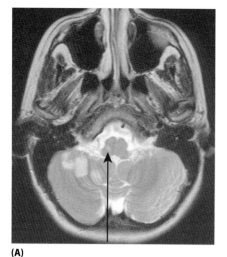

(A)

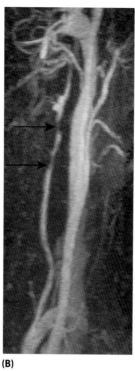

(B)

Fig. 5 **Vertebral artery dissection shown at magnetic resonance imaging.** (A) Note the infarcts within the cerebellar hemisphere and within the medulla (arrow), emphasizing the sensitivity of MR imaging. (B) MR angiogram of the cervical vertebral artery showing the irregular contour caused by arterial dissection (arrows).

Thromboembolism

Up to 80% of ischaemic strokes result from thromboembolism from atheromatous disease at the carotid bifurcation. If the stenosis is severe, then carotid endarterectomy or, possibly, stenting will be necessary in carefully selected patients in an attempt to prevent further stroke (Fig. 6). With lesser degrees of stenosis, medical therapy with anti-platelet drugs, such as aspirin, is preferred. Ultrasound of the carotid arteries is usually the first line of vascular imaging, increasingly followed by MR or possibly CT angiography, rather than invasive and somewhat hazardous catheter angiography in this group (Fig. 7).

Cerebral venous occlusion

Ischaemic strokes can also arise from cerebral venous occlusion. The typical scenario is that of a young female, a few weeks post partum, who develops convulsions, focal neurological signs and, in the most severe cases, becomes comatose. Imaging shows haemorrhagic infarcts and dural venous sinus thrombosis.

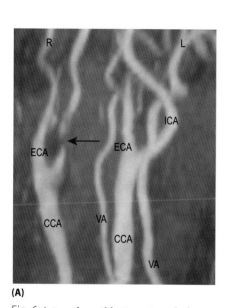

(A)

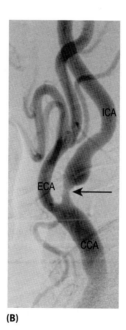

(B)

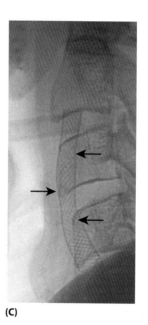

(C)

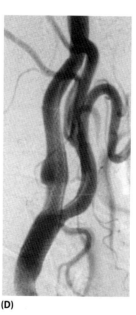

(D)

Fig. 6 **Internal carotid artery stenosis demonstrated at magnetic resonance angiography.** (A) Stenosis is shown in the right internal carotid artery (ICA) (arrow). The ICA on the left is normal. VA, vertebral artery; CCA, common carotid artery; ECA, external carotid artery. (B) Lateral view from a selective common carotid angiogram demonstrating the internal carotid artery stenosis (arrow). (C) Following stent insertion. (D) After contrast injection.

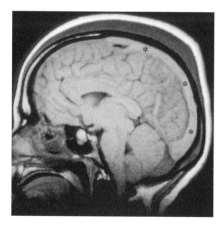

Fig. 7 **Dural venous sinus thrombosis.** The sagittal cranial magnetic resonance image shows thrombosis of the superior sagittal sinus (*).

> ## Ischaemic stroke
>
> - The majority of strokes are ischaemic.
> - Thromboembolism from the cervical carotid bifurcation or from the heart is the usual cause.
> - Computed tomography is the initial investigation of choice, but may be normal for 24 hours of cerebral ischaemia.

Cerebral haemorrhage

Spontaneous intraparenchymal haemorrhage, into the brain proper, is often associated with hypertension (as with ischaemic stroke). The typical hypertensive haemorrhage is situated in the basal ganglia (Fig. 1) and causes a hemiparetic stroke, which is difficult, if not impossible, to distinguish clinically from one due to ischaemia. Hypertensive haemorrhage can also affect the brainstem.

If a haematoma is large, its mass effect will cause raised intracranial pressure and may require urgent surgical evacuation.

Haemorrhage is very simple to identify on computed tomography (CT), accounting for its primary role in the initial management of acute cerebral conditions, both traumatic and non-traumatic. There will be evidence of haemorrhage on the initial scan unlike the situation with ischaemia, which may take 12–24 hours to appear. The representation of haemorrhage on magnetic resonance imaging (MRI) is much more complex because of the several blood products each contributing to the signal at different times during evolution of the clot. Chronic haemorrhage (weeks to months old) is typically high signal (white) due to the methaemoglobin on T1- and T2-weighted images (Fig. 2), with a surrounding signal void (black) due to haemosiderin seen better on T2. The evidence of haemorrhage also persists far longer on MRI (several months or even years) than CT (a few days only) (see p. 102).

If the clinical picture and CT findings are typical of an hypertensive haemorrhage then no further imaging may be undertaken, but one is always alert to an underlying cause for a cerebral haemorrhage, which might be caused by either a cerebral arteriovenous malformation (AVM) or neoplasm. An AVM is an abnormal collection of arteries and veins, without an intervening capillary bed (Fig. 3). It is probably a congenital abnormality but presents only rarely in childhood. Patients present from the third decade onwards with haemorrhage, epilepsy, headache or progressive neurological deficit. The

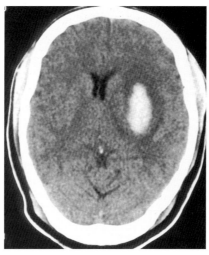

Fig. 1 **A computed tomography scan showing hypertensive haemorrhage** in the basal ganglia.

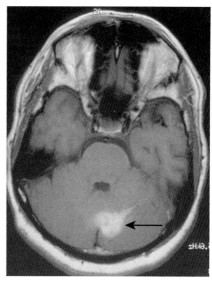

Fig. 2 **Cerebellar haemorrhage** (arrow) demonstrated on a T1-weighted magnetic resonance sequence.

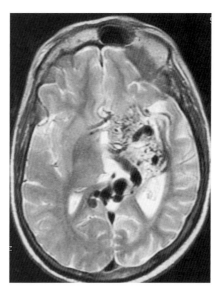 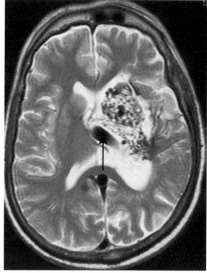

Fig. 3 **Cerebral arteriovenous malformation.** Magnetic resonance imaging shows multiple, black 'signal voids'. These represent vessels, the larger ones being the draining veins (arrow).

last occurs when the high blood flow through the AVM 'steals' blood from the normal brain. MRI and catheter angiography will be necessary to evaluate an AVM and the neuroradiologist may undertake embolization to reduce the size of an AVM before surgical excision or radiotherapy (Fig. 4).

The cavernous angioma or cavernoma is another type of vascular malformation occurring within the brain. It can give rise to epilepsy or it may bleed, and it may be multiple. Occasionally it may be inherited. Cerebral angiography is normal, leading to the alternative term of 'angiographically occult vascular

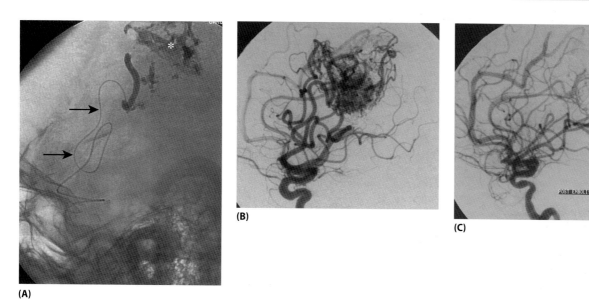

(A)

(B)

(C)

Fig. 4 **Embolization of an arteriovenous malformation (AVM).** (A) The microcatheter (arrows) is seen within an intracranial artery supplying the AVM. A mixture of 'superglue' and opacifying agent has been injected into the AVM 'nidus' or centre (*). (B and C) Carotid angiogram. Lateral views obtained before (B) and after (C) the embolization shown in (A).

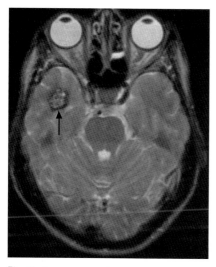

Fig. 5 **Cavernous angioma.** The axial T2-weighted MRI shows a typical cavernoma in the right temporal lobe.

malformation'. The MRI appearances are however characteristic and angiography is seldom necessary. The cavernoma consists of a black rim ('signal void'), due to haemosiderin surrounding a white ('high signal') centre consisting of methaemoglobin (Fig. 5). The signal change is consistent on both T1- and T2-weighted images. Cavernomas are lobulated and their shape serves to distinguish them from simple haemorrhage.

To identify what are usually more aggressive primary tumours and some metastases associated with haemorrhage, it may be appropriate to rescan after an interval when the haemorrhage has regressed. It is usually the case, however, that tumour is not completely enveloped by haemorrhage and can thus be recognized.

> ## Cerebral haemorrhage
>
> - Cerebral haemorrhage can give rise to a stroke syndrome indistinguishable from a cerebral infarct.
> - An underlying cause for the haemorrhage should be considered.
> - Computed tomography is the initial investigation of choice.

Subarachnoid haemorrhage

Spontaneous subarachnoid haemorrhage (SAH) usually results from the rupture of a berry aneurysm, most of which are borne on the arterial circle of Willis at the base of the brain (Fig. 1). Forty per cent of aneurysms arise on the anterior cerebral arteries, 30% on the internal carotid artery, 22% on the middle cerebral artery and 8% on the vertebral and basilar arteries. The major arteries supplying the brain, including the

circle, are situated in the subarachnoid space, which contains cerebrospinal fluid (CSF). Along the inferior surface of the brain there is a number of interconnecting and relatively capacious CSF 'cisterns'. The circle of Willis is in the suprasellar cistern above the pituitary gland. Aneurysmal haemorrhage, in the first instance, therefore, mixes with the CSF and produces a severe headache with nausea, vomiting and neck stiffness.

Haemorrhage can rupture into the cerebral ventricles causing intraventricular haemorrhage with hydrocephalus. This may be due either to blood causing obstruction to the flow of CSF within the ventricles or to a failure of CSF resorption by the arachnoid granulations.

Aneurysmal rupture can also result in haemorrhage into the brain (intracerebral haemorrhage) and, occasionally, into the subdural space (subdural haematoma).

This is a very serious condition, commoner in females, the outcome of which is approximately thus: one-third die, one-third are disabled and one-third do well. Medical treatment is directed towards combating the effects of the haemorrhage on the brain, notably arterial vasospasm leading to cerebral ischaemia. Surgical treatment to the aneurysm is undertaken in order to prevent recurrent bleeding, the peak incidence of which occurs in

the first 2 weeks after the first rupture. Of course, hydrocephalus and a life-threatening intracerebral haematoma may also require surgical intervention.

Imaging of a patient with suspected subarachnoid haemorrhage

Computed tomography

The clinical suspicion of SAH is investigated in the first instance with cranial computed tomography (CT), which can both confirm the diagnosis and identify the likely site of the aneurysm responsible (about 20% of patients will subsequently be shown to have two or more aneurysms).

The visibility of the subarachnoid blood on CT will depend both on the amount of bleeding and the time interval between the haemorrhage and the scan. In a typical case, blood mixed with CSF turns the normally dark basal cisterns white (Fig. 2). The likely position of a ruptured aneurysm is more accurately identified if it is associated with an intraparenchymal haemorrhage (Fig. 3).

The 'white' blood will fade over time and there may not be a large amount in the first place. **It is, therefore, axiomatic that a 'normal' CT scan does not exclude SAH.** In this case, the CSF must be examined to exclude the diagnosis.

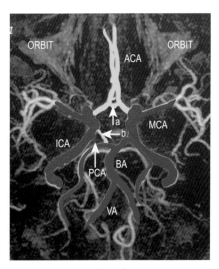

Fig. 1 **Normal examination.** Axial MR angiogram showing the circle of Willis. a, anterior communicating artery; b, posterior communicating artery; ACA, anterior cerebral arteries; MCA, middle cerebral artery; ICA, internal carotid artery; BA, basilar artery; PCA, posterior cerebral artery; VA, vertebral artery.

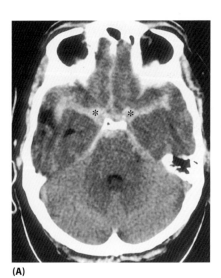

(A)

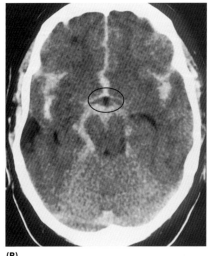

(B)

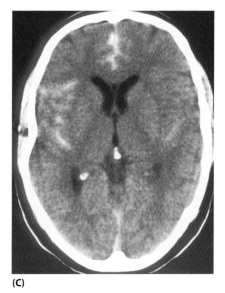

(C)

Fig. 2 **Subarachnoid haemorrhage.** (A) The computed tomography scan shows a white 'blood' cisternogram (*). (B and C) The oval outlines the optic chiasm and the posterolaterally directed optic tracts within the suprasellar cerebrospinal fluid cistern.

It is not uncommon for the patient's condition to deteriorate before or following surgical treatment, and CT will be required to identify the possible causes, including recurrent haemorrhage, hydrocephalus or vasospastic cerebral ischaemia. Vasospasm occurs most commonly between 3 and 13 days after subarachnoid haemorrhage, and it may be appropriate to operate early before the onset of vasospasm if the patient is relatively well.

Use of magnetic resonance imaging, especially FLAIR sequences

Magnetic resonance imaging (MRI) is relatively insensitive to subarachnoid haemorrhage and is not used routinely in the management of these patients. Nevertheless, patients with SAH may be directed to MRI, if the diagnosis is not clear-cut. The FLAIR (**FL**uid **A**ttenuated **I**nversion **R**ecovery) sequence may be useful, as the only MRI pulse sequence to demonstrate SAH reliably (Fig. 4).

Angiography

Although catheter angiography remains the gold standard for the pre-operative evaluation of aneurysms, MR angiography and, particularly, CT angiography are being used increasingly.

Interventional radiology

Endovascular neuroradiological techniques are rapidly replacing the surgical clipping of aneurysms. Using fine microcatheters, platinum coils are inserted into the aneurysm sac to pack it as much as possible and provoke thrombosis to obliterate the sac and prevent further bleeding (Fig. 5).

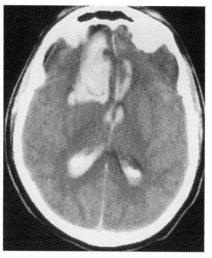

Fig. 3 **Rupture of an anterior communicating artery aneurysm.** Computed tomography demonstrates haemorrhage into the medial frontal lobe and ventricular system.

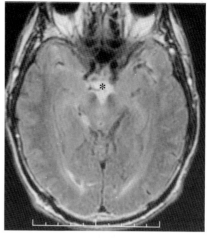

Fig. 4 **Subarachnoid haemorrhage** (*) is shown on an axial MR FLAIR sequence.

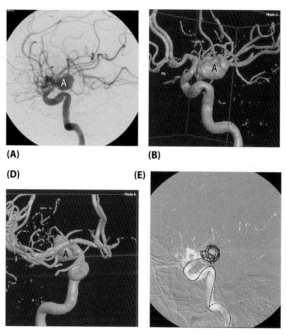

(A)   (B)   (C)

(D)   (E)

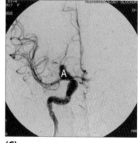

Fig. 5 **Coil embolization of an internal carotid artery aneurysm** (A) arising at the origin of the posterior communicating artery. (A and B) Lateral conventional and 3-D angiographic views. (C and D) Frontal conventional and 3-D angiographic views. (E) A platinum coil is shown being positioned within the aneurysm sac through a microcatheter.

Subarachnoid haemorrhage

- Computed tomography (CT) is the imaging investigation of choice for the diagnosis of subarachnoid haemorrhage and its complications.
- CT can indicate the location of the responsible aneurysm.
- A normal CT scan does not exclude subarachnoid haemorrhage.

Intracranial tumours 1

Intracranial tumours can be divided into those which are intra-axial (or intrinsic) and extra-axial (or extrinsic).

Intra-axial tumours

Intra-axial tumours arise in the brain proper and are usually malignant to a greater or lesser degree. They are classified on the basis of cell-type and graded according to various histological indicators of malignancy (Box 1). The most malignant is the glioblastoma multiforme (Fig. 1).

Calcification within a primary intrinsic tumour points towards a less aggressive tumour and contrast enhancement usually, though not always, to a more malignant process. It should be appreciated, however, that an initially indolent tumour can become aggressive and, therefore, calcification may be found within a highly malignant primary tumour.

Cerebral tumours can be primary or metastases can spread to the brain from

> ### Box 1 *Intracranial tumours*
>
> **Intra-axial (arising within the brain)**
> Gliomas
> - Astrocytoma
> - Oligodendroglioma
> - Ependymoma
> - Ganglioglioma.
>
> Primitive neuroectodermal tumour (PNET)
> Primary lymphoma
> Metastases (but some can be extra-axial, e.g. from breast or prostate primaries).
>
> **Extra-axial (intracranial but extracerebral)**
> Meningioma
> Pineal region tumours
> Tumours from cranial nerves, e.g. acoustic neuroma
> Chordoma
> Craniopharyngioma
> Epidermoid
> Dermoid.

elsewhere. The brain is a recognized site for metastases from carcinomas of the lung or breast and from malignant melanoma. Oedema can be a feature of benign as well as malignant tumours. Although the distinction may be difficult, a metastasis usually has a large amount of oedema and a primary tumour relatively little in comparison to the tumour mass (Fig. 2). It should be remembered, however, that the 'oedema' surrounding an enhancing primary neoplasm may contain tumour cells. Multiple lesions naturally suggest metastases, but gliomas can sometimes be multifocal.

As a rule, primary brain tumours do not metastasise outside of the neuraxis (brain and spinal cord). They can, however, spread via the cerebrospinal fluid (CSF) in the subarachnoid space, resulting in 'seeding' of tumours, which can involve the brain, cord or meninges (Fig. 3).

An intrinsic tumour of the cerebellum in an adult is a metastasis until proven otherwise. Primary tumours, nevertheless, occur in this region (Fig. 4), and the brainstem and cerebellum are the commonest sites for cerebral tumours in children (Fig. 5).

von Hippel-Lindau disease is inherited as an autosomal dominant trait and is associated with multiple haemangioblastomas occurring in the cerebellum, spinal cord and retina. Affected individuals are also at risk from phaeochromocytomas, renal cell carcinoma and cysts of the liver, pancreas and kidney.

Tumours may also arise within the ventricles from the ependymal lining (Fig. 6) and from the choroid plexuses, which secrete CSF. Interestingly, meningiomas may also be intraventricular.

Tuberous sclerosis is another condition associated with cerebral tumours. Along with neurofibromatosis (see p. 114) it is one of the neurocutaneous syndromes with skin and central nervous system manifestations. It can be inherited as an autosomal dominant trait but more often occurs spontaneously. Affected individuals suffer mental retardation and seizures.

Within the brain arise a variety of abnormalities, including cortical tubers

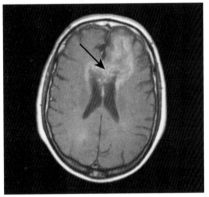

(A)

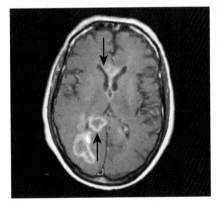

(B)

Fig. 1 **Glioblastoma multiforme** – axial magnetic resonance sequence after intravenous gadolinium DTPA. (A and B) This highly malignant and peripherally enhancing tumour involves both hemispheres, spreading across the corpus callosum (arrows). This is the largest of the commissural tracts which, by definition, connect the hemispheres.

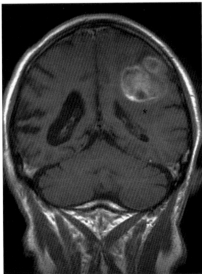

Fig. 2 **Malignant glioma.** This T1-weighted coronal MRI scan after intravenous gadolinium DTPA shows the enhancing tumour in the parietal lobe. There is relatively little surrounding oedema (*).

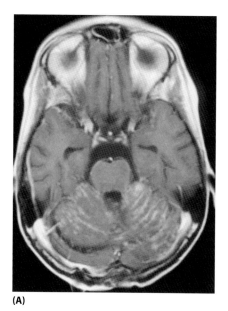

(A)

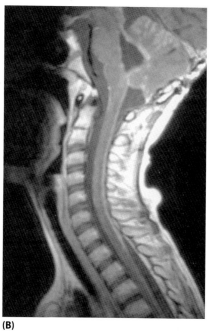

(B)

Fig. 3 **Metastases from medulloblastoma.** Axial cranial (A) and sagittal spinal (B) magnetic resonance images after intravenous gadolinium DTPA. The metastases have resulted in 'sugar coating' of the brain and spinal cord.

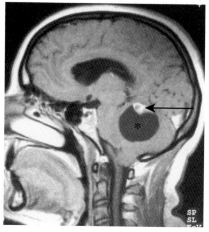

Fig. 4 **Cystic cerebellar haemangioblastoma (*).** This sagittal magnetic resonance sequence following intravenous injection of gadolinium DPTA shows an enhancing mural nodule (arrow). These appearances are very similar to a cystic astrocytoma.

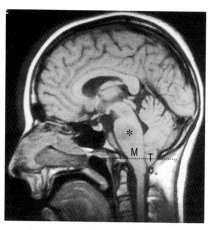

Fig. 5 **Pontine glioma** (*) – sagittal magnetic resonance image. The pons is swollen and there is mass effect with both the cerebellar tonsils (T) and medulla (M) displaced inferiorly below the foramen magnum (dotted line).

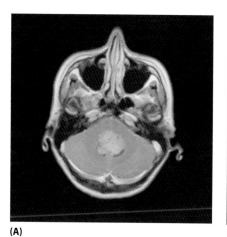

(A)

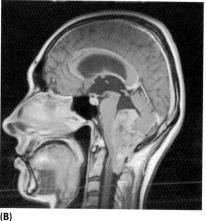

(B)

Fig. 6 **Ependymoma** – axial (A) and sagittal (B) magnetic resonance images following intravenous gadolinium DTPA. The tumour has arisen within the fourth ventricle and has extended through the foramen of Magendie into the spinal subarachnoid space.

and subependymal nodules, both of which may calcify. In particular the condition is associated with giant cell astrocytomas in the region of the foramen of Monro, which links the lateral and third ventricles (Fig. 7). These tumours are generally indolent but may cause obstructive hydrocephalus with lateral ventricular enlargement.

Intracranial tumours 1

- Intracranial tumours can be intra-axial or extra-axial. Intra-axial tumours are usually malignant; extra-axial tumours are usually benign.
- Primary tumours of the neuraxis only rarely metastasise outside of the central nervous system.
- Intra-axial tumours of the cerebellum in an adult are metastases until proven otherwise.
- Computed tomography and magnetic resonance imaging cannot distinguish reliably between tumoral recurrence or post radiotherapy effects.

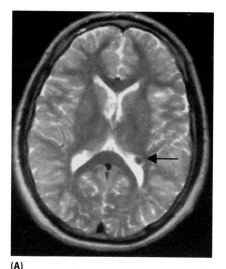

(A)

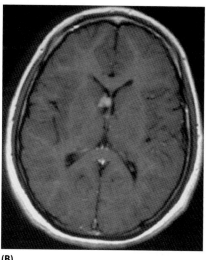

(B)

Fig. 7 **Tuberous sclerosis.** The T2-weighted axial image (A) shows a subependymal nodule (arrow). The T1-weighted axial image (B) after intravenous gadolinium DTPA reveals an enhancing giant cell astrocytoma near to the foramen of Monro.

Intracranial tumours 2

Extra-axial tumours

Extra-axial tumours are intracranial but extracerebral and are usually benign (see Box 1 for intra- and extra-axial tumours). A typical example is the meningioma, arising from the dura mater investing the brain and lining the inner skull vault and base.

Meningioma

Tumours arising from the meninges are the most common intracranial tumours. They are generally well-defined and cause symptoms by a pressure effect on the underlying brain. They do not generally invade the brain substance, but often invade the skull, causing a local periosteal reaction with a 'hair-on-end' or destructive pattern. The venous sinuses are often invaded. Meningiomas occur in the region of the sagittal sinus, the sphenoid bone and also around the pituitary fossa. They occur in middle-aged or elderly females and have fairly characteristic imaging appearances (Figs 1 & 2).

Some 15% of these lesions calcify and, in addition, erosion of the adjacent skull may be present, so that changes may be seen on a plain film in 30% of patients.

Acoustic neuroma

The acoustic neuroma arises from the vestibular division of the vestibulocochlear (VIII) cranial nerve, within the internal auditory canal and grows into the posterior fossa (Fig. 3). There is an association with neurofibromatosis, a heritable mesodermal dysplasia, when bilateral tumours may be encountered as well as neuromas and other tumours elsewhere in the neuraxis.

There are two variants of neurofibromatosis, NF-1 and NF-2, both of which are inherited.

NF-1 patients may have a variety of skin lesions, notably café-au-lait spots and soft, fleshy neurofibromas. They are also prone to generally slow growing gliomas affecting the optic pathway and elsewhere in the cerebral hemispheres and cerebellum.

The pathognomonic feature of the less common NF-2 is bilateral acoustic neuromas. Patients may also develop neuromas of the other cranial nerves and spinal nerve roots. There is also an increased incidence of meningiomas.

Figure 3 shows the typical features of an extra-axial tumour.

The acoustic neuroma arises from the vestibulocochlear (VIII) cranial nerve in the internal auditory canal and, while clearly separate from it, compresses and displaces the brain (Fig. 3).

The acoustic neuroma is the commonest tumour (90%) occurring in the cerebellopontine angle (between pons, cerebellum and the medial aspect of the petrous temporal bone). Meningiomas are the next commonest, then epidermoid tunours a distant third.

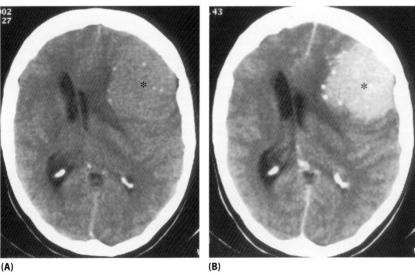

(A)　　　　　　　　　　**(B)**

Fig. 1 **Meningioma** – cranial computed tomography scans before (A) and after (B) intravenous iodinated contrast medium. This tumour (*) shows flecks of calcification and has a broad base against the inner skull vault, which is lined by dura from which the meningioma originates. Note the mass effect.

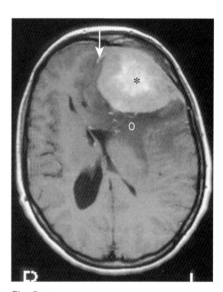

Fig. 2 **Meningioma** (same patient as Fig. 1) – axial magnetic resonance image after intravenous gadolinium DTPA. Note the dural tail (arrow), which is a typical, though not exclusive, feature. There is also low signal oedema (O) around the tumour.

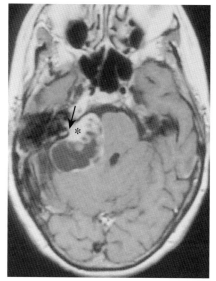

(A)

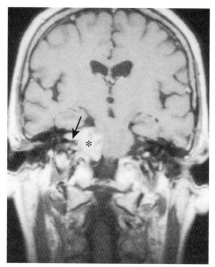

(B)

Fig. 3 **Acoustic neuroma** (*) arising from the vestibulocochlear (VIII) cranial nerve in the internal auditory canal (arrow). (A) Axial and (B) coronal magnetic resonance images after intravenous gadolinium DTPA. This is a typical example of an extra-axial tumour of the vestibulocochlear (VIII) cranial nerve.

Imaging of intracranial tumours

The radiologist's functions after identification of a potential tumour are to characterize it as far as possible, to localize it anatomically and to identify any pressure effects such as hydrocephalus and or herniation. With the exception of calcification, all these requirements are better met with magnetic resonance imaging (MRI).

The presence of a mass lesion or cerebral swelling from any cause can lead to significant mass effect, hydrocephalus and cerebral herniation. Herniation involves the movement of structures from one cerebral compartment to another. The compartments are partitioned by relatively inelastic dura against which compression occurs. There can be shift across the midline under the falx cerebri, the incomplete dural partition between the cerebral hemispheres. The falx is sickle-shaped and thinner anteriorly, where midline shift is thus more pronounced (see Fig. 2).

Mass effect can be exerted downwards with impaction at the foramen magnum (see Fig. 5, p. 113). The most serious effects of mass are when the brainstem is compressed when potentially fatal 'coning' occurs.

It can prove difficult to distinguish tumour from an infective mass on imaging alone, particularly when a mass lesion has a cyst-like component, and, in the majority of cases, biopsy or surgical resection are undertaken.

After therapy, imaging is necessary to confirm the excision of a benign tumour or to monitor the progress of a malignant tumour. The changes due to radiotherapy can mimic tumour recurrence exactly on MRI or computed tomography (CT), and it may be necessary to resort to positron emission tomography (PET) scanning or MR spectroscopy to make the distinction.

Intracranial tumours 2

- Magnetic resonance imaging (MRI) is the imaging modality of choice.
- It can be difficult to distinguish a tumour from an infective mass on imaging alone.
- Changes due to radiotherapy can mimic tumour recurrence on MRI or computed tomography.
- Positron emission tomography scanning or MR spectroscopy can be used to identify tumour recurrence after surgery and radiotherapy.

Pituitary gland and perisellar region

The pituitary gland is situated within the descriptively named sella turcica (Turk's saddle) or pituitary fossa on the superior surface of the body of the sphenoid bone in the central skull base (Fig. 1). It secretes a variety of hormones, mainly trophic, from its anterior and posterior lobes. The normal pituitary gland should measure no more than 10 mm in height in women of reproductive age, although the upper limit of normal increases to 12 mm in late pregnancy and post partum. The superior margin of the gland may also be convex in these groups.

The pituitary stalk or infundibulum, part of the posterior lobe, extends superiorly and a little posteriorly towards the hypothalamus. Just anterior to the stalk is the optic chiasm and, also superior to the gland, within the suprasellar cerebrospinal fluid (CSF) space ('cistern'), is the arterial circle of Willis. On either side of the gland are the cavernous sinuses. These are extradural venous spaces through which the third (oculomotor), fourth (trochlear) and sixth (abducent) cranial nerves pass to supply the extraocular muscles. The ophthalmic (V1) and maxillary (V2) divisions of the fifth (trigeminal) nerve and the internal carotid arteries also traverse these sinuses.

Beneath the pituitary fossa, the pneumatized sphenoid body (the sphenoid air sinus) facilitates the pernasal, trans sphenoidal surgical approach to the gland.

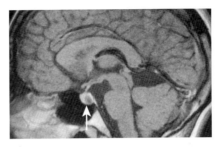

Fig. 2 **Pituitary microadenoma** (arrow). Sagittal magnetic resonance image after intravenous gadolinium DTPA.

Tumours of the pituitary gland

A variety of tumours arise within the pituitary gland. A proportion of small tumours (**microadenomas**) are discovered incidentally (20%), but those that present clinically do so because of the effects of hormonal overproduction (Fig. 2). The commonest is the **prolactinoma** (30%). Prolactin-secreting tumours, which are commoner in females, result in galactorrhoea, amenorrhoea and infertility.

A tumour producing growth hormone causes **pituitary gigantism** if it arises before puberty and **acromegaly** if it develops later in life. **Cushing's disease** (as distinct from Cushing's syndrome) results from a pituitary adenoma causing excess corticosteroid production.

Imaging of the pituitary gland

The pituitary gland is best imaged with magnetic resonance imaging (MRI). Microadenomas are shown as small mass lesions within the gland, often with only minimal disturbance to its overall size and shape. The pituitary gland does not have a blood–brain barrier so that it enhances with intravenous contrast agents – gadolinium (Gd)-DTPA for MRI and various iodinated agents for computed tomography (CT).

The unenhanced MR image may not show an abnormality other than gland enlargement but after MRI contrast enhancement with Gd-DTPA administration, the adenoma will either fail to enhance significantly or, if

a dynamic series of scans is obtained, enhance more slowly than the normal gland. Cushing's adenomas are notoriously difficult to identify on imaging, and hormonal assays on venous blood draining from the cavernous sinuses may be necessary to lateralize the tumour (petrosal sinus sampling).

Developmental cysts
Non-functioning, developmental cysts (Rathke's cleft cysts) may also occur, which can sometimes attain a substantial size.

Macroadenoma
The larger tumours, which are often 'non-functioning', are usually macroadenomas and may cause compressive effects on adjacent structures, notably the optic pathway, immediately superior to the pituitary gland. The classical visual field defect described when the optic chiasm is compressed is bitemporal hemianopia. These tumours may also precipitate pituitary failure, which can occur acutely, even in small tumours, if haemorrhage occurs. The typical macroadenoma with suprasellar extension takes on an hour-glass shape particularly in the coronal plane, its waist constricted by the dural diaphragma sellae, which forms the roof of the fossa (Fig. 3). The pituitary fossa is also expanded or 'ballooned'.

Extension of a pituitary tumour laterally into the cavernous sinuses can cause an ophthalmoplegia, but cavernous sinus invasion may prove difficult to identify with imaging. If anything, it tends to be over-diagnosed.

Meningioma
Meningiomas are the second commonest tumours of this region and arise within the cavernous sinus or from the skull base adjacent to the pituitary fossa (Fig. 4). Extension anteriorly from the cavernous sinus towards the optic canal may result in visual loss. They normally have a broad base and may calcify, belying their dural origins. Pituitary tumours rarely calcify and in the presence of a meningioma the pituitary gland can be identified separately.

Pathology affecting the posterior pituitary usually results in a loss of function, that is, diabetes insipidus (DI).

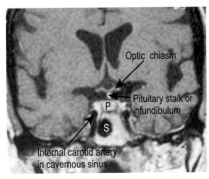

Fig. 1 **Normal study.** Coronal magnetic resonance image after gadolinium DTPA. P, pituitary gland; S, sphenoid air sinus.

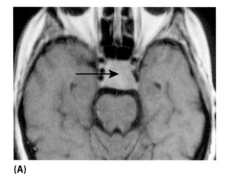

(A)

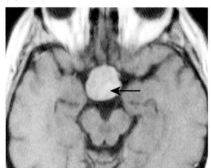

(B)

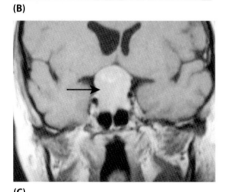

(C)

Fig. 3 **Pituitary macroadenoma** (arrow). Axial (A and B) and coronal (C) magnetic resonance images after intravenous gadolinium. The uniformly enhancing mass expands the pituitary fossa and extends superiorly to occupy the suprasellar cerebrospinal fluid cistern, where it compresses the optic chiasm (not shown).

Craniopharyngioma

Craniopharyngioma is the commonest of the suprasellar tumours and may cause DI, precocious puberty or visual impairment. There are two peaks of incidence, between 5 and 15 years, and between 50 and 60 years. It has calcific and cystic elements and will show enhancement, unlike developmental cysts. Again the pituitary gland should be definable separate from the tumour, although meningiomas and craniopharyngiomas can be intrasellar.

Should a patient with known malignancy develop DI, then a pituitary metastasis should be sought.

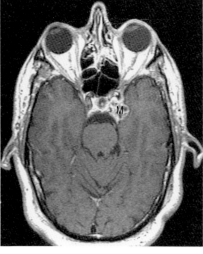

Fig. 4 **Cavernous sinus meningioma** (M). Axial magnetic resonance image after intravenous gadolinium DTPA. An enhancing tumour is shown.

Aneurysm

The third commonest perisellar 'mass' is an aneurysm (Fig. 5). These can arise from the internal carotid artery within the cavernous sinus, producing painful ophthalmoplegia. However, those that are entirely within the sinus do not result in subarachnoid haemorrhage if they rupture, rather a caroticocavernous arteriovenous fistula. However, an arterial aneurysm large enough to mimic a pituitary tumour can develop near to the midline from the circle of Willis and this may rupture into the subarachnoid space.

The identification of a sellar mass lesion as an aneurysm is, of course, crucial prior to treatment but usually, in practice, not difficult. There are pulsation artefacts visible on MRI and evidence of blood flow through the aneurysm and of blood products should there be partial thrombosis.

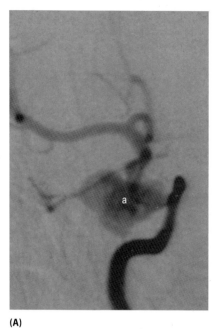

(A)

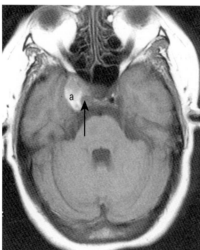

(B)

Fig. 5 **Cavernous aneurysm.** (A) The aneurysm (a) is shown on the frontal view at angiography. (B) Axial magnetic resonance image. The arrow points to the occluded carotid artery, performed therapeutically.

Pituitary gland and perisellar region

- Pituitary tumours present when small, due to hormonal over-production, the commonest being prolactinomas.

- Large pituitary tumours may also be hormone-secreting but often present as a result of optic pathway compression. Cavernous sinus invasion can also occur with ophthalmoplegia.

- Craniopharyngiomas, meningiomas and aneurysms occur in the sellar and perisellar regions.

Hydrocephalus

Hydrocephalus is defined as 'dilatation of the cerebral ventricular system'. It is associated with a variety of developmental (congenital) abnormalities (Fig. 1), or it may result from intrauterine infection with rubella, cytomegalovirus or toxoplasmosis (Box 1). It may also be acquired later in life.

The formation of adhesions can result in hydrocephalus after pyogenic meningitis and it is a common consequence of tuberculous meningitis. Hydrocephalus may also follow subarachnoid haemorrhage or trauma. These processes usually result in global ventricular enlargement (Table 1).

Box 1 Classification of hydrocephalus

Communicating hydrocephalus (failure of cerebrospinal fluid resorption)
Congenital infection
Meningitis
Head injury
Subarachnoid haemorrhage.

Non-communicating or obstructive hydrocephalus
Congenital
  ■ Aqueduct stenosis
  ■ Chiari malformation
  ■ Dandy Walker syndrome.
Acquired
  ■ Tumours or haemorrhage (both intraventricular or parenchymal)

Over-production of CSF
Choroid plexus papilloma

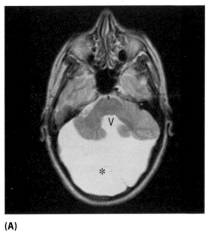

(A)

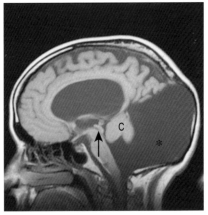

(B)

Fig. 1 **Dandy Walker cyst** (*) – axial (A) and sagittal (B) magnetic resonance images. There is a large cyst in the enlarged posterior cranial fossa associated with maldevelopment of the cerebellum (C) and an absent vermis. The fourth ventricle (V) opens into the cyst. The arrow points to the cerebral aqueduct.

Obstructive hydrocephalus

Cerebrospinal fluid (CSF) is formed in the choroid plexuses, situated within the cerebral ventricles. Out of a total volume of about 125 ml, 25 ml are within the ventricles, the remainder within the craniospinal subarachnoid space. CSF flows from lateral to third to fourth ventricles and out into the subarachnoid spaces. It is absorbed into the venous circulation by the arachnoid granulations near to the superior sagittal sinus. As a result of this circulation, 50% is replaced every 5–6 hours. The site of an obstructing mass lesion, which may not be immediately obvious on a scan, can be predicted on the basis of CSF circulation. The part of the system 'upstream' of the obstruction will be dilated, the part 'downstream' will remain normal (Figs 2 & 3).

An obstruction within the ventricles results in 'non-communicating' hydrocephalus and when outside, for instance, when the arachnoid granulations are involved in post-inflammatory adhesions, the hydrocephalus is termed 'communicating'. In communicating hydrocephalus, all the ventricles will be enlarged, although the fourth is often only marginally dilated.

Obstructive hydrocephalus must be differentiated from the ventricular dilatation that accompanies the volume loss of cerebral atrophy and that is far commoner in adults. It may not always be an easy distinction, but in atrophy the temporal horns of

---

Table 1 **Causes of hydrocephalus**				
Site of obstruction	**Causes**	**Lateral ventricle**	**Third ventricle**	**Fourth ventricle**
Foramen of Monro	Colloid cyst Tumour, e.g. giant-cell Astrocytoma	Enlarged	Normal	Normal
Cerebral aqueduct	Congenital Midbrain or pineal region tumour Adhesions from haemorrhage or infection	Enlarged	Enlarged	Normal
Fourth ventricular 'outflow' (foramina of Magendie and Luschka)	Tumour in cerebellum, brainstem or 4th ventricle Adhesions from haemorrhage or infection	Enlarged	Enlarged	Enlarged
Extraventricular obstruction ('communicating' hydrocephalus)	Congenital Adhesions from haemorrhage or infection	Enlarged	Enlarged	Normal or enlarged

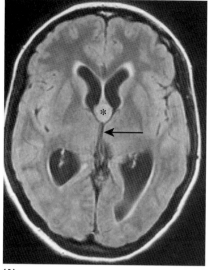

(A)

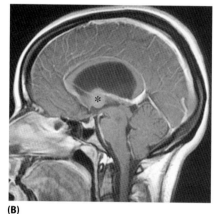

(B)

Fig. 2 **Colloid cyst of the third ventricle** (*) – axial (A) and sagittal (B) magnetic resonance images. These cysts obstruct the foramen of Monro which connects the lateral and third ventricles. The slit-like third ventricle (arrow) thus remains normal in size.

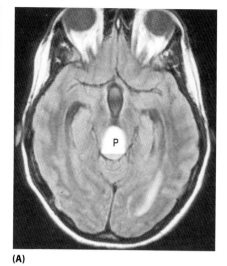

(A)

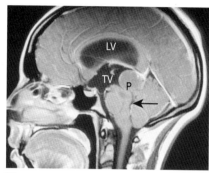

(B)

Fig. 3 **Pineal cyst** (P) – axial (A) and sagittal (B) magnetic resonance images. The pineal gland is related to the posterior part of the third ventricle. The cerebral aqueduct in the midbrain, which connects the third and fourth ventricles, is obstructed. This has led to dilatation of the lateral (LV) and third (TV) ventricles, but has spared the fourth, which is compressed (arrow).

neurological deficit). Imaging is not diagnostic but large ventricles are present. Distinction from atrophy can be difficult and CSF pressure monitoring, may be required. CSF pressure is raised intermittently and the condition is thus incorrectly described.

Imaging following treatment

Treatment is directed at removing the underlying cause, where possible, and draining the CSF, either temporarily with external ventricular drainage or permanently with a 'shunt'. The shunt device consists of a tube, fitted with a valve mechanism to prevent reflux, which leads from the cerebral ventricle to the cardiac atrium or the peritoneum.

Initial drainage must be controlled to prevent subdural haematomas, which arise if decompression is too rapid. CT scanning after drainage is used to verify the correct position of the tube, which must avoid the highly vascular choroid plexus, and to monitor the reduction in ventricular size. Clinical deterioration may result from shunt malfunction, in which case plain radiographs are used to check the integrity of the shunt, or subdural haematoma formation. On occasion, CSF can form an extracerebral collection, called a subdural hygroma.

the lateral ventricles usually remain near-normal in size. Particularly in children, CSF may cross the ependymal lining of an obstructed ventricle and enter the surrounding white matter, resulting in periventricular low density on computed tomography (CT) and equivalent signal change on magnetic resonance imaging (MRI).

'Normal-pressure' hydrocephalus

One particular entity worthy of note is 'normal-pressure hydrocephalus'. This is a somewhat poorly understood condition affecting the elderly. Affected patients have the classic triad of dementia, incontinence and gait dyspraxia (the inability to undertake purposive movement in the absence of

Hydrocephalus

- Hydrocephalus may result from obstruction to cerebrospinal fluid (CSF) flow either within the ventricular system (non-communicating hydrocephalus) or outside of it.

- The site of obstruction can be deduced from knowledge of CSF flow.

- Normal pressure hydrocephalus affects the elderly, causing dementia, gait dyspraxia and urinary incontinence.

Multiple sclerosis

Multiple sclerosis (MS) is an inflammatory condition, of unknown cause, in which plaques of demyelination occur in the white matter of brain and spinal cord. It is typically a relapsing-remitting condition affecting young adults and with a female preponderance. The presentations are varied, but patients may develop visual failure due to retrobulbar neuritis, various sensory disturbances or paraparesis, when the spinal cord is involved.

Imaging of multiple sclerosis

In all but the most advanced cases computed tomography (CT) is normal.

Magnetic resonance imaging (MRI) is the investigation of choice and, indeed, is the only imaging method that can be relied on to demonstrate the lesions of MS.

Magnetic resonance imaging
The typical appearance on cerebral T2-weighted or FLAIR MRI consists of multiple ovoid lesions in the white matter surrounding the cerebral ventricles (Fig. 1). The lesions have their long axes in a radial distribution, reflecting inflammation around medullary veins that radiate outwards from the lateral ventricles (Fig. 2). There is also a predilection for the corpus callosum, which may atrophy selectively (Fig. 3), and the middle

cerebellar peduncle. Active plaques may be surrounded by some oedema and may enhance with intravenous gadolinium DTPA. Rarely, the lesions in MS can be large and even haemorrhagic, resembling a tumour (tumorous MS). Indeed, one of the differential diagnoses of a large enhancing juxtaventricular lesion is lymphoma.

Differential diagnosis between multiple sclerosis and other conditions

Acute disseminated encephalomyelitis
The imaging findings in MS may be indistinguishable from the much less common acute disseminated encephalomyelitis (ADEM), which is a

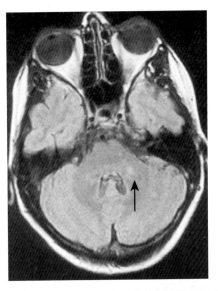
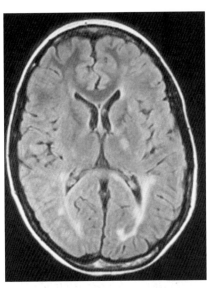
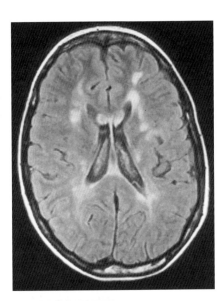

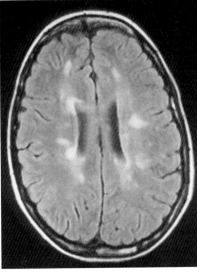
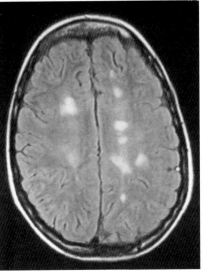

Fig. 1 **Multiple sclerosis** – series of axial magnetic resonance scans – FLAIR sequence. Numerous ovoid lesions are seen within white matter. A lesion is seen within the middle cerebellar peduncle (arrow).

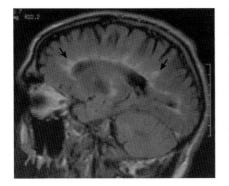

Fig. 2 **Multiple sclerosis.** The FLAIR sagittal MR sequence demonstrates the radial distribution of the plaques of demyelination (arrows).

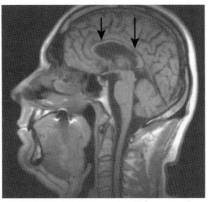

Fig. 3 **Multiple sclerosis** – sagittal magnetic resonance image. Atrophy of the corpus callosum (arrows).

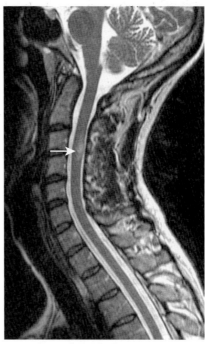

Fig. 4 **Multiple sclerosis** – sagittal T2-weighted magnetic resonance image. A plaque of demyelination is shown in the cervical cord (arrow).

monophasic illness characteristically occurring after a viral infection or vaccination.

Small vessel ischaemic change
The more usual distinction the radiologist is required to make on MRI is between MS and so-called 'small vessel ischaemic change' in the brain (see Fig. 4, p. 106). Ischaemic lesions are seen within the basal ganglia, unlike MS. In the periventricular white matter they are irregular in both size and shape, unlike the ovoid shape and radial distribution of MS. Callosal and peduncular lesions favour MS. The differentiation can be difficult and the 'end stages' of both conditions can be identical with atrophy and generalized, confluent white-matter signal change.

It is probable that all patients with MS have plaques in the spinal cord, but MRI is less sensitive to their presence (Fig. 4). Usually they appear on T2-weighted images as high signal lesions within the cord, the contour of which is normal or nearly normal. Local swelling and enhancement can sometimes occur, superficially resembling a cord tumour. As with the brain, advanced disease can cause atrophy of the cord (Fig. 5).

After the initial diagnosis, subsequent MR imaging can be used to monitor disease activity and assist in therapy.

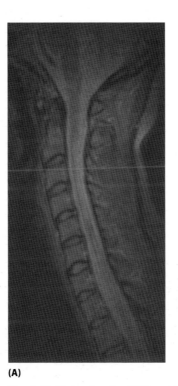
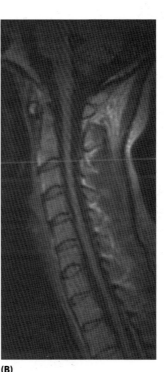

(A) **(B)**

Fig. 5 **Multiple sclerosis.** (A) T2- and (B) T1-weighted MR sequences show multiple lesions within an atrophied cervical spinal cord (compare with Fig. 4).

Multiple sclerosis

- In multiple sclerosis (MS), magnetic resonance imaging (MRI) is the investigation of choice.
- Small vessel ischaemic change may resemble MS on MRI.
- MS is the commonest cause of lesions found within the spinal cord on MRI.

Craniospinal injury

Blunt head injuries may be caused by direct impact and inertial injury, alone or in combination. Primary injury occurs at the time of impact. Secondary effects are delayed and include infection, hydrocephalus, arterial damage and, in the worst cases, focal or generalized atrophy. Head injuries may be open or closed, depending on whether brain and meninges are exposed to the exterior, but it should be appreciated that serious cerebral injury can occur in the absence of a skull fracture.

Contusions of the brain

Cerebral injury may be in the form of contusions or bruises, which are relatively superficial and can be found in the inferior frontal and temporal lobes in relation to the irregular contour of the adjacent inner surface of the skull (Fig. 1).

Diffuse axonal injury

Diffuse axonal injury (DAI) is thought to result from shearing injury, that is, the differential movement of one part of the brain relative to others, but it should be emphasized that the causative mechanisms in the various lesions in head injury may not be entirely clear. Lesions in DAI may or may not be haemorrhagic, typically occurring in the corpus callosum,

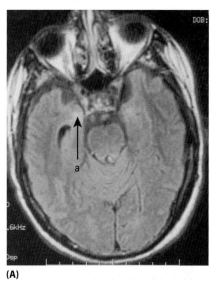

(A)

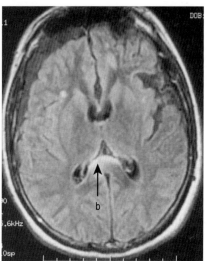

(B)

Fig. 2 **Diffuse axonal injury (DAI).** (A) DAI affects the uncus (a) and corpus callosum. (B) The corpus callosum (b) is affected. Scattered white matter lesions are also shown.

basal ganglia, grey-white cortical junction and upper brainstem. Magnetic resonance imaging (MRI) may be particularly valuable in this condition (Fig. 2).

Extra-axial haemorrhage

Two types of extra-axial haemorrhage may be found, the incidence of which is far greater in the presence of a skull fracture. These occupy spaces or potential spaces between the inner surface of the skull and the brain.

The **extradural** haemorrhage usually results from damage to the middle meningeal vessels underlying a

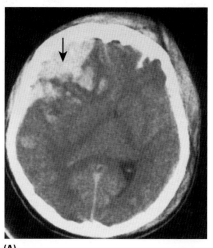

(A)

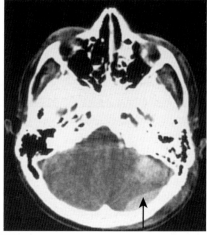

(B)

Fig. 3 **Extradural haemorrhage** seen on axial computed tomography scanning (A) in the frontal region (arrow) and (B) in the posterior fossa (arrow). Note also the cerebral contusions. The lesions are biconvex in shape.

temporal bone fracture, but can occur elsewhere (Fig. 3). It is biconvex in shape and almost always presents acutely.

The **subdural** haematoma is crescentic in shape and, if acute, is associated with severe cerebral injury (Fig. 4). Subdural haematomas may also present as a chronic lesion and may be bilateral. Chronic subdural haematomas occur in the very young and in the elderly. In babies they are part of the clinico-radiological spectrum of 'non-accidental injury' (see p. 100). In the elderly they may present with intellectual deterioration and progressive hemiparesis similar to a tumour. Hence, the value of axial scanning in this latter group to identify a treatable cause.

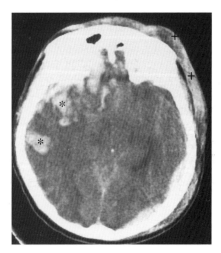

Fig. 1 **Acute haemorrhagic contusion.** The axial computed tomography scan shows changes in the inferior frontal and temporal lobes (*) due to contusion. The site of impact is on the opposite side (+). This is a contrecoup injury.

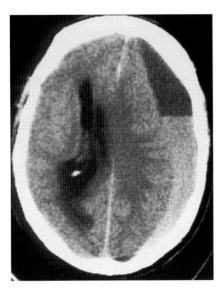

Fig. 4 **Subdural haematoma** seen on axial computed tomography scanning. Patients are scanned in the supine position. There has been layering of the blood products with a fluid-fluid level, the denser (brighter) elements lying inferiorly.

Imaging of head injury

The central investigation in head injury is cranial computed tomography (CT), because of its ability to demonstrate the various types of haemorrhage allied to the convenience and simplicity of the examination. The role of skull radiography has remained somewhat controversial. However, it is the intracranial compartment that is of primary interest. A digital radiograph of the skull is acquired as part of the cranial CT and the axial images can be viewed on bone 'settings' to look for fractures. These may not disclose undisplaced fractures parallel to the axial scan plane, but are far superior in the detection of fractures of the skull base.

Perhaps the major problem involves those with ostensibly minor head injury. Should they have a skull series of plain radiographs, since a fracture is known to be associated with an increased risk of an extra-axial collection? It is well known that, in practice, the actual number of fractures seen is very low. One may resort then to a clinical approach, discharging the patient with instructions to carers to use a head injury 'chart', describing, in lay terms, clinical features which warrant re-examination. If the patient is incapacitated through alcohol or drugs, there may be a lower threshold to performing a cranial CT.

Non-accidental injury
MRI is useful in non-accidental injury (see also p. 100) where it is important to identify injuries that have occurred at separate times. Subdural haematomas are rare in children and if they are found in the absence of significant accidental trauma or, more commonly, with an unconvincing explanation from the carers, non-accidental injury (NAI) should be suspected. Because of the facility of MRI to track the evolution of haematoma, it can be used to confirm that the bilateral subdural haematomas are different ages.

Spinal injury in association with head injury
Spinal injury often accompanies accidental head injury, but is not a common association in non-accidental injury. The cervical column, being mobile, is most vulnerable and is subject to a variety of fractures, dislocations and ligamentous injuries. Patients with severe craniospinal injuries, after a preliminary plain film series, often undergo CT scanning of the vertebral column at the same time as a cranial CT to minimize potential harm to the patient during transportation. Less severe cases or conscious patients can be assessed clinically, but broadly CT is used to assess bony injury; MRI is used for the soft tissues especially the spinal cord (Fig. 5).

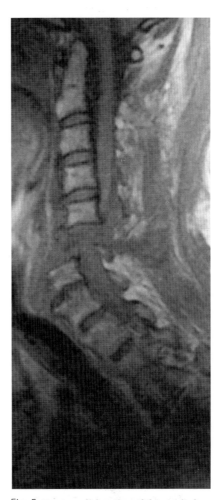

Fig. 5 **Fracture-dislocation of the cervical spine with transection of the cord** seen on sagittal magnetic resonance imaging.

Craniospinal injury

- Computed tomography (CT) is the initial investigation in head injury.
- Head and spinal injury often co-exist.
- Bilateral subdural haematomas in children should alert clinicians to the possibility of non-accidental injury.
- In the vertebral column, after plain film examination, CT is the investigation of choice to characterize fractures. Magnetic resonance imaging is used to examine the spinal cord, intervertebral discs and ligaments.

Craniospinal infection 1

Meningitis

Cranial imaging has little part to play in the diagnosis of suspected acute bacterial or viral meningitis, the former normally part of a septicaemia. Imaging will be necessary particularly in *recurrent* meningitis when it is mandatory to search either for a local source of infection, such as within the petrous bone or paranasal sinuses or for a portal of entry for the organisms. Following a basal skull fracture, for instance, leakage of cerebrospinal fluid (CSF) may occur (CSF rhinorrhoea or otorrhoea), which may require surgical closure. Thin-section coronal computed tomography (CT) is used on occasion, with iodinated contrast agent introduced into the CSF via lumbar puncture.

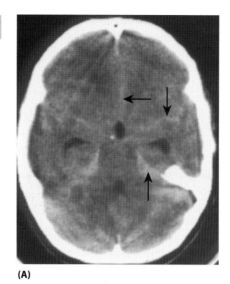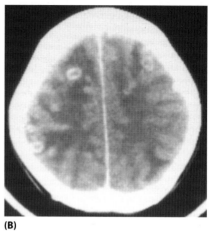

(A)   **(B)**

Fig. 1 (A and B) **Tuberculous meningitis and multiple tuberculomas** – cranial computed tomography scan following intravenous iodinated contrast medium. There is basal meningitis with enhancement (arrows). Multiple ring-enhancing intracerebral tuberculomas are also present.

Tuberculosis

Cranial tuberculosis gives rise to a granulomatous meningitis, usually with hydrocephalus. Magnetic resonance imaging (MRI) or CT show enhancement of the basal meninges (MRI more sensitively) and there may also be intracranial lesions ('tuberculomas') (Fig. 1). These are solid or, more characteristically, ring-enhancing lesions surrounded by varying amounts of oedema and mass effect.

Pyogenic infection and abscess formation

Pyogenic infection may also lead to a cerebral abscess. Again, it is important to identify a local source of infection. Otogenic abscesses, due to ear infection, characteristically occur either within the cerebellum or temporal lobe, both of which are related to the petrous bone. The paranasal sinuses may be responsible or septic emboli can involve the brain from an extracranial source.

A cerebral abscess is typically a ring-enhancing lesion arising at the grey-white-matter junction (Fig. 2). On occasion, the abscess can rupture into the cerebral ventricle.

It is important to appreciate that an abscess can resemble a cerebral

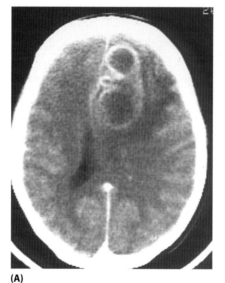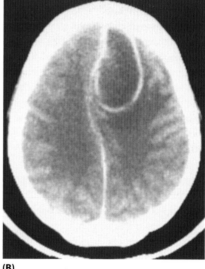

(A)   **(B)**

Fig. 2 (A and B) **Cerebral abscess** – axial computed tomography scan after intravenous iodinated contrast medium. The patient had cyanotic congenital heart disease, a recognized though rare association of cerebral abscess.

tumour so that it may not be possible to make a distinction, particularly in the absence of the typical systemic features of infection. This is one reason why intracerebral mass lesions are biopsied, even those where the likelihood of tumour is high.

Cranial infection involving the paranasal sinuses or petrous temporal bone can result in the formation of subdural or, less commonly, extradural empyemas. They may also be a complication of surgery and/or trauma. Both can be classed as extra-axial lesions in much the same way as neoplasms. A cerebral abscess is an intra-axial lesion.

Subdural empyemas form over the cerebral surface or in the interhemispheric fissure. Since infection can spread via the cerebral veins, the collections may be some way

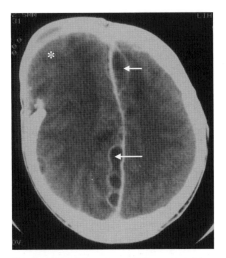

Fig. 3 **Subdural empyema (abscess).** Axial-computed tomography scan after intravenous iodinated contrast medium. Note the loculated collections adjacent to the falx cerebri (arrows). Note the frontal lobe herniating through the defect (*) after surgical removal of the overlying skull vault to 'decompress' the swollen brain.

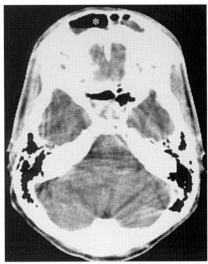

(A)

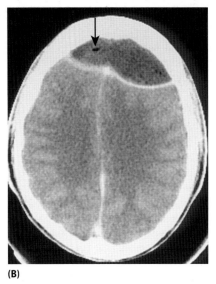

(B)

Fig. 4 (A and B) **Extradural abscess due to frontal sinusitis** – axial computed tomography scan after intravenous iodinated contrast medium. Note the air-fluid level in the frontal sinus (*) and the air within the abscess (arrow) due to a breach in the wall of the sinus.

from the source of infection and are often multiple (Fig. 3). They may be difficult to identify on CT even after intravenous iodinated contrast medium, and MRI is the more sensitive examination.

An extradural empyema is usually next to the source, with direct spread from the paranasal sinus, petrous bone or calvarial osteomyelitis (Fig. 4).

Treatment of intracranial or cerebral infection is generally urgent and usually requires a combination of surgical drainage and antibiotic therapy, with attention also paid to the source of infection.

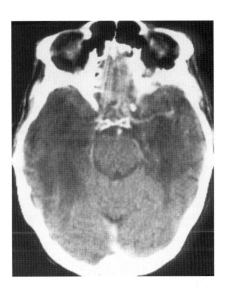

Fig. 5 **Herpes simplex encephalitis** – cranial computed tomography scan after intravenous iodinated contrast medium. This severe case shows symmetrical low density (attenuation) in both temporal lobes.

Encephalitis

MRI is the investigation of choice in suspected viral encephalitis owing to its greater sensitivity in the detection of early parenchymal change in comparison to CT. Herpes simplex encephalitis, the commonest variety of this rare condition, has a predilection for the temporal and, to a lesser extent, the frontal lobes (Fig. 5).

Craniospinal infection 1

- In the diagnosis of acute, uncomplicated, pyogenic or viral meningitis, imaging has little part to play.

- It may not be possible to differentiate cerebral abscess and tumour on magnetic resonance imaging or computed tomography. Hence, surgical biopsy or excision are frequently performed.

- Suspected intracranial infection is an emergency.

Craniospinal infection 2: HIV/AIDS and spinal infection

HIV/AIDS and superadded infections

Cerebral changes in HIV/AIDS can result from effects of the virus itself or from superadded infections, such as toxoplasmosis, progressive multifocal leukoencephalopathy (PML) and cryptococcosis. Tuberculosis and syphilis may also occur. Primary lymphoma is the cerebral tumour most associated with, but not unique to HIV/AIDS.

HIV is neurotropic and can lead to rapidly progressive cerebral atrophy and diffuse white-matter change.

Toxoplasmosis

This typically manifests as a ring-enhancing lesion in the basal ganglia. There may be several lesions (Fig. 1).

Lymphoma

This can be difficult to distinguish from toxoplasmosis. It too can be multifocal, but, in general, it occurs close to the cerebral ventricles (Fig. 2).

Progressive multifocal leukoencephalopathy

This is due to a papova virus and leads to patchy, asymmetrical white-matter abnormality, seen much better on magnetic resonance imaging (MRI) than on computed tomography (CT) (Fig. 3). Progressive multifocal leukoencephalopathy (PML) is the most common manifestation of cerebral AIDS in children. Both toxoplasmosis and lymphoma are uncommon in the paediatric AIDS population.

Cryptococcosis

This is a fungal disease, which, on MRI, gives rise to basal ganglia and midbrain changes with the formation of cyst-like lesions. The perivascular spaces also become dilated and a meningeal component to the disease may give rise to contrast enhancement.

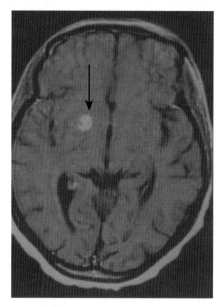
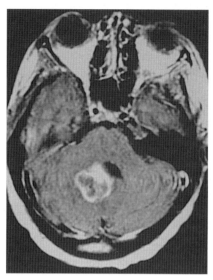

Fig. 1 **Toxoplasmosis in an adult patient with HIV/AIDS.** Two enhancing lesions are seen on the T1-weighted axial magnetic resonance image following intravenous gadolinium DPTA. The basal ganglia lesion (arrow) is typical, but these appearances may also be found in lymphoma.

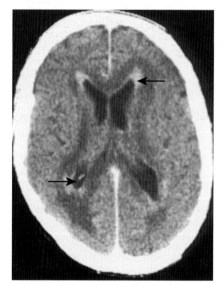
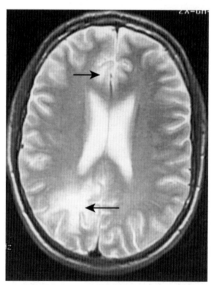

Fig. 2 **Cerebral lymphoma** – axial computed tomography scan after intravenous iodinated contrast medium. Enhancing tumour (arrows) with oedema (low attenuation) is seen close to the cerebral ventricles.

Fig. 3 **Progressive multifocal leukoencephalopathy (PML)** in a patient with HIV/AIDS – T2-weighted axial magnetic resonance sequence. The asymmetric white-matter lesions (arrows) are a characteristic feature.

Meningitis may affect the entire neuraxis, that is, brain and spinal cord, but infection of the vertebral column usually involves the relatively avascular intervertebral discs extending to the vertebrae as an osteomyelitis.

Spinal infection (see also p. 12)

Pyogenic discitis can be part of a septicaemic illness, but is most commonly encountered as a complication of lumbar discal surgery (Fig. 4). Tuberculosis also involves disc spreading to adjacent bone, but more often in the thoracic column (Fig. 5). It seems a more destructive process than pyogenic infection, leading to vertebral collapse, the formation of epidural

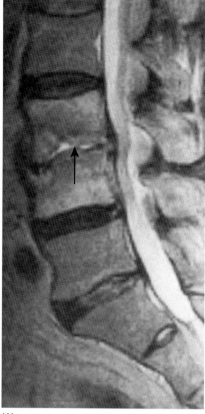

(A)

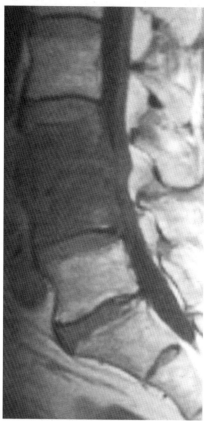

(B)

Fig. 4 **Lumbar discitis following discal surgery.** Note the narrowed disc on the sagittal T2-weighted magnetic resonance sequence (arrow) and oedema of the vertebral bodies, shown as bright signal on the T2-weighted image (A) but dark on T1-weighting (B).

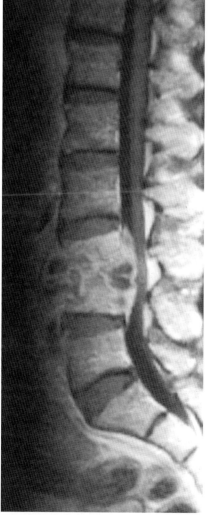

(A)

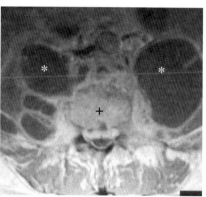

(B)

Fig. 5 **Tuberculosis of the spine with psoas abscesses.** (A) The sagittal magnetic resonance (MR) image shows destruction of the disc between L3 and L4, with fusion of these two vertebral bodies. They too are partially destroyed. There is a large posterior spinal mass compressing the canal, spinal theca and spinal roots. (B) Axial MR images show the ghostly outline of the abnormal post-infective vertebral body (+) and large paraspinal soft-tissue masses. The central low signal dark areas within these masses are the psoas abscesses containing pus (*). The walls of the abscesses enhance after intravenous gadolinium and appear bright.

soft-tissue masses and abscesses within the psoas muscles. In both pyogenic and tuberculous infection of the vertebral column, bony collapse, fusion and spinal deformity may be the final result.

Craniospinal infection 2

Cerebral infection in HIV/AIDS
- The brain is involved in up to 40% of patients with HIV/AIDS, due to HIV itself, superadded infections or tumour.

Spinal infection
- Discitis is most commonly seen as a complication of lumbar discal surgery.

Myelopathy

Lesions of the vertebral column, which may result in progressive myelopathy and/or compression of the spinal cord, are conveniently classified according to their anatomical location.

Extradural lesions

Extradural lesions, the commonest, and usually originating in bone, include degenerative disease and metastatic infiltration (Fig. 1A). Trauma will be considered separately.

Intradural extramedullary lesions

Less common are the intradural extramedullary, such as neurofibromas and meningiomas, arising within the dura but separate from the spinal cord (Fig. 1B).

Intramedullary lesions

Least common of all are the intramedullary lesions (Fig. 1C), arising within the spinal cord, and are usually inflammatory (multiple sclerosis), a syrinx cavity or tumours (Fig. 1C).

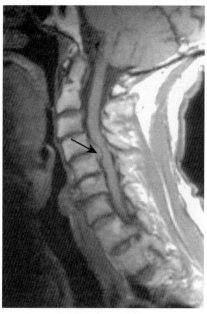

Fig. 2 **Cervical spondylosis and disc protrusion causing spinal cord compression.** The sagittal T1-weighted magnetic resonance sequence shows that the discs are reduced in height and that there is malalignment of the vertebrae. A very large dorsal discal protrusion is compressing the cord at C4/5 level (arrow).

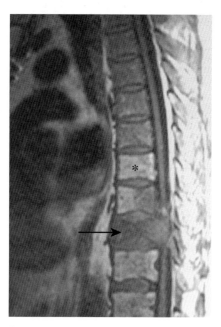

Fig. 3 **Metastatic disease of a thoracic vertebral body** – T1-weighted magnetic resonance (MR) image. MRI is very sensitive to change in the bone marrow, particularly T1-weighted sequences. The normal fatty (yellow) marrow (*) is replaced by darker tumour (arrow). The vertebral body has collapsed with tumour entering the spinal canal, causing spinal cord compression.

Degenerative joint disease of the spine

Degenerative disease, in the form of cervical spondylosis, can lead to paraparesis or quadriparesis with cord compression resulting from large

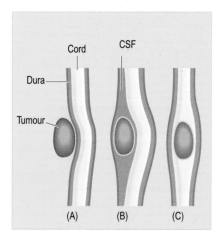

Fig. 1 **Differentiation** between (A) extradural, (B) intradural extramedullary and (C) intramedullary mass lesions.

osteophytes projecting posteriorly into the spinal canal. Usually, though not always, in younger adults, a disc protrusion may be responsible (Fig. 2). Similarly, both spondylosis and a disc protrusion can lead to a compressive radiculopathy (of an exiting nerve root) and can, therefore, cause upper or lower motor neurone disorder, either alone or in combination. Symptomatic degenerative disease is far less common in the thoracic column and, in the lumbar region, almost always causes cauda equina (lower motor neurone) compression.

Metastatic bone disease

Metastatic infiltration of bone leading to vertebral collapse and cord compression can occur anywhere in the vertebral column, but is most often found in the thoracic region (Fig. 3). Metastases can occur in any of the three compartments mentioned, but

are progressively less common as one moves 'inwards'.

Tumours and other lesions

Neurofibromas arise from nerve roots either sporadically or as part of von Recklinghausen's neurofibromatosis (NF-1). The tumours expand the intervertebral canals, in which they arise, and often extend both within the spinal canal and outside of the column as a 'dumb bell' tumour (Fig. 4).

Intrinsic tumours of the spinal cord are rare, but include ependymoma and astrocytoma (Fig. 5).

Vascular malformations and infarction of the cord may also be encountered, but inflammatory lesions, usually due to multiple sclerosis, are far commoner (see p. 120).

A syrinx, or fluid-filled cavity, in the spinal cord usually occurs in

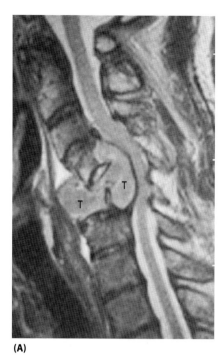

(A)

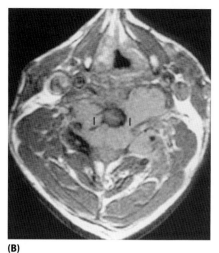

(B)

Fig. 4 **Neurofibromatosis.** (A) The sagittal magnetic resonance (MR) image demonstrates that the tumour (T) has eroded bone and caused vertebral collapse. Cord compression results. (B) The axial MR sequence shows that this large tumour has also extended through and eroded the intervertebral foramina (I).

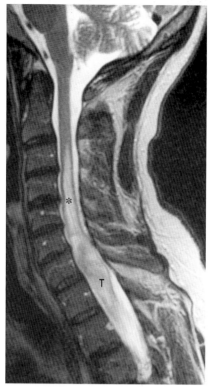

Fig. 5 **Intrinsic spinal cord tumour** (T) – sagittal T2-weighted magnetic resonance image of the cervical spine. There is cord oedema superiorly (*).

association with congenital descent of the cerebellar tonsils which disturbs normal cerebrospinal fluid circulation (Fi.g 6).

Investigation of myelopathy

The imaging investigation of myelopathy centres on magnetic resonance imaging (MRI), which is the only investigation to demonstrate parenchymal change within the spinal cord due to myelitis, infarct, trauma or tumour.

MRI will readily localize a mass lesion into one or other of the spinal 'compartments' described above. The multiplanar facility allows the entire vertebral column to be surveyed in suspected metastatic disease.

It may, of course, be necessary to perform cranial MRI to aid diagnosis, notably in suspected multiple sclerosis, or to assess the extent of malignancy affecting the neuraxis.

Unless there is a contraindication to MRI, computed tomography (CT) myelography is, at most, an adjunct. It is, however, useful in characterizing bone disease.

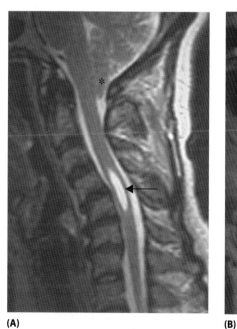

(A)

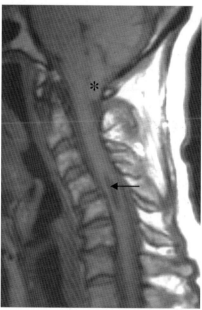

(B)

Fig. 6 **Syrinx within the cervical spinal cord** (arrow). The (A) T2- and (B) T1-weighted MRI sequences also show descent of the cerebellar tonsils (*) below the foramen magnum.

Myelopathy

■ Most conditions resulting in myelopathy are extradural in type and arise from bone. Degenerative disease of the cervical spine is the commonest.

■ Metastatic disease usually affects the vertebral column. Meningeal involvement is less common. A metastasis to the spinal cord is rare.

■ Intrinsic tumours of the spinal cord are rare. Inflammatory lesions of the spinal cord, often multiple, as part of multiple sclerosis are far commoner.

Index

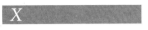